EXPLORING
THE PSYCHOLOGY, DIAGNOSIS, AND TREATMENT OF
NEUROGENIC COMMUNICATION DISORDERS

DENNIS C. TANNER, PH.D.

iUniverse, Inc.
New York   Bloomington

Exploring the Psychology, Diagnosis, and Treatment of Neurogenic Communication Disorders

The information, ideas, and suggestions in this book are not intended as a substitute for professional medical advice. Before following any suggestions contained in this book, you should consult your personal physician. Neither the author nor the publisher shall be liable or responsible for any loss or damage allegedly arising as a consequence of your use or application of any information or suggestions in this book.

iUniverse books may be ordered through booksellers or by contacting:

iUniverse
1663 Liberty Drive
Bloomington, IN 47403
www.iuniverse.com
1-800-Authors (1-800-288-4677)

Because of the dynamic nature of the Internet, any Web addresses or links contained in this book may have changed since publication and may no longer be valid. The views expressed in this work are solely those of the author and do not necessarily reflect the views of the publisher, and the publisher hereby disclaims any responsibility for them.

ISBN: 978-1-4502-1376-9 (sc)
ISBN: 978-1-4502-1377-6 (dj)
ISBN: 978-1-4502-1378-3 (ebk)

Printed in the United States of America

iUniverse rev. date: 06/04/2010

Table of Contents

Part II: The Psychology of Neurogenic Communication Disorders

Introduction

Exploring the Psychology, Diagnosis, and Treatment of Neurogenic Communication Disorders is written for those seeking an advanced examination of these oftentimes devastating disorders. Whether the reader is a student, clinician, scientist, or a family member of the patient, this book provides current, relevant, and important information about aphasia, apraxia of speech, dysarthria, and the communication disorders associated with traumatic brain injury. This text also examines important psychological aspects of these disorders including depression, anxiety, psychosis, loss and grief, and impaired psychological defense mechanisms and coping styles which occur in many patients.

This book is the culmination of more than three decades of my research, teaching, and clinical management of neurogenic communication disorders. Neurogenic communication disorders are often controversial clinical entities, sometimes passionate topics of discussion, and never unimportant to students, scientists, clinicians, and family members of the patient. By bringing together the important scientific and clinical issues in one text, I believe the reader will be stimulated, educated, and enlightened about these communication disorders which can have dramatic effects on quality of life for patients and their families.

Dennis C. Tanner, Ph.D.
January 8, 2010

About the Author

Dennis C. Tanner received the Doctor of Philosophy degree in Audiology and Speech Sciences from Michigan State University. Professor Tanner's books include *The Family Guide to Surviving Stroke and Communication Disorders* (2nd ed.); *The Psychology of Neurogenic Communication Disorders: A Primer for Health Care Professionals; Exploring Communication Disorders: A 21st Century Introduction Through Literature and Media; Case Studies in Communication Sciences and Disorders; An Advanced Course in Communication Sciences and Disorders; The Forensic Aspects of Communication Sciences and Disorders; The Medical-Legal and Forensic Aspects of Communication Disorders, Voice Prints, and Speaker Profiling; Case Studies in Dysphagia Malpractice Litigation;* and *On Neurogenic Communication Disorders: Original Short Stories and Case Studies.* He is also the coauthor of the *Quick Assessment Series for Neurogenic Communication Disorders.* Dr. Tanner has been named Outstanding Educator by the Association of Schools of Allied Health Professions, and has been the College of Health Profession's Teacher of the Year. He serves as an expert witness in legal cases involving communication sciences and disorders and is currently Professor of Health Sciences at Northern Arizona University in Flagstaff, Arizona. For more information, visit his website: www.drdennistanner.com

Part I

The History, Nature, Etiology, Diagnosis, and Treatment of Neurogenic Communication Disorders

Chapter One: Introduction to Neurogenic Communication Disorders

"The most incomprehensible thing about the
world is that it is at all comprehensible."

Albert Einstein

Chapter Preview: In this textbook, neurogenic communication disorders are broadly defined to include the language disorder of aphasia, the motor speech disorders of apraxia of speech and the dysarthrias, certain neurogenic perceptual impairments, and the communication disorders associated with traumatic brain injury. There is also an overview of gross neuroanatomy as it pertains to neurogenic communication disorders. The psychology of neurogenic communication disorders and quality of life issues are also discussed.

Communication Disorders Resulting from Neurologic Injury

Of the multitude of diseases, defects, disorders, and disabilities afflicting humans, few can be as devastating as neurogenic communication disorders. Certainly, some communication disorders resulting from neurologic injury can simply be inconveniences and have little effect on the patient's overall quality of life. For example, minor strokes and temporary palsies can be insubstantial impairments to a person's ability to communicate effectively, and to deal with day-to-day family, work, and social activities. The communication disorders arising from these minor and temporary medical conditions are more nuisances than life-altering barriers to quality living. Of course, there are individual differences in the way people deal with medical adversity and what is only minor and inconvenient to one person may be altogether devastating to another. However, as a rule, most people deal appropriately and proportionally with medical adversity and minor and temporary neurogenic communication disorders are minimally disruptive to their overall quality of life.

> "Communication disorders will be a major public health concern for the 21st century because, untreated they adversely affect the economic well-being of a communication-age society" (Ruben, 2000, pg. 245).

Unfortunately, minor and temporary neurogenic communication disorders are rare. Most neurogenic communication disorders are significant in magnitude and chronic, if not permanent. Some neurogenic communication disorders come on suddenly. For example, in stroke-related neurogenic communication disorders, there is no time for the patient to prepare for the medical emergency, and nearly instantly, he or she loses some or all of the ability to communicate. Other neurogenic communication disorders develop slowly, such as those resulting from progressive degenerative neuromuscular diseases. Initially, the symptoms are barely noticeable, but overtime, they can render the person completely unable to speak, write, or gesture meaningfully. Neurogenic communication disorders associated with traumatic brain injuries occur violently and are often associated with major behavioral, cognitive, and emotional changes. Communication impairments and irregularities are sometimes frightening initial symptoms of Alzheimer's disease and other dementias, and foretell the wasting of mental functions to follow.

While not minimizing the human devastation that can be caused by neurogenic communication disorders, this broad class of speech, voice, and language disorders is interesting to study. For scientists and clinicians alike, the research and academic study of these communication disorders are challenging and thought-provoking. Research and academic study of neurogenic communication disorders transcend several complex disciplines such as human anatomy and physiology, neurology, psychiatry, psychology, and neuropsychology. The normal cognitive, neurological, and psychological substrates of language and motor speech production are the highest and most evolved function of which humans are capable, and we have barely scratched the surface in understanding them. And with incomplete understanding of the normal process of language and motor speech production, clinicians are charged with evaluating and treating the multitude of communication disorders resulting from neurologic damage. The scientific and academic study of neurogenic communication disorders, and the treatment of patients suffering from them, is an exciting yet challenging endeavor for scientists and clinicians.

Definition of Neurogenic Communication Disorders

> According to Rubin (2000), the prevalence of all communication disorders ranges between 5% and 10% and cost the United States between $154 and $186 billion annually.

Neurogenic communication disorders are speech, voice, and language disorders arising from damage to the brain and nervous system. In this text, a broad definition of neurogenic communication disorders is used to encompass aphasia, motor speech disorders, and the speech pathologies and language deficits associated with traumatic brain injury. This all encompassing definition of neurogenic communication disorders addresses the following diagnostic categories of communication disorders:

Aphasia: An acquired loss or disruption of language due to damage to the major speech and language centers of the brain. Aphasia is the multimodality inability to encode, decode, and manipulate symbols for the purposes of verbal thought and/or communication.

Apraxia of Speech: The impaired ability to conceptualize, program, and execute voluntary neuromuscular speech movements.

Agnosia: A perceptual disorder involving the difficulty recognizing and appreciating information coming from the senses and usually specific to one modality of communication.

Dysarthrias: A general category of neuromuscular disorders resulting from damage to the brain and nervous system. The dysarthrias affect, more or less, the timing, strength, range of motion, speed, and appropriateness of motor speech movements.

Language of Confusion: Language reflecting reduced or impaired consciousness often associated with traumatic brain injury.

Each of the above categories of neurogenic communication disorders will be discussed, described, and further defined in subsequent chapters of this book. Additionally, the specific neurological and muscular anatomic and physiologic factors associated with each category of communication disorders will be provided. However, to understand neurogenic communication disorders, examining the general human nervous system is necessary.

Gross Neuroanatomy

Although the nervous system functions as a whole, it is divided into the *peripheral* and *central systems.* Twelve *cranial nerves,* 31 pairs of spinal nerves, and the autonomic nervous system make up the peripheral nervous system. The brain and spinal cord comprise the central nervous system and both are covered by the three protective membranes collectively known as the *meninges.* The outermost membrane is the *dura mater* and the innermost membrane is the *pia mater.* Found between the two is a weblike membrane known as the *arachnoid mater.* "A space between the arachnoid and pia mater is filled with cerebrospinal fluid, which enters the space from the fourth ventricle and circulates around the brain and spinal cord" (Zemlin, 1998, p. 325). The peripheral nervous system senses changes in the body or external environment and conveys that information to the central nervous system. The central nervous system reacts to that input and sends signals back to the peripheral nervous system. The central nervous system has more redundancy, but the peripheral system tends to regenerate damaged neurons.

Brain Hemispheres

The brain weights about 3 pounds and contains more than twenty billion nerve cells. Connected by the *corpus callosum*, the brain is divided into two hemispheres. The hemispheres consist of an outer layer of *cerebral cortex* which is between 1.25-4.0 mm thick, an intermediate mass of white matter fibers, and an inner mass of gray matter fibers called the *basal nuclei* (Culbertson, Cotton, and Tanner, 2006). In most persons, the left hemisphere is dominant for speech and language functions. The right hemisphere is also involved in simple speech and language functioning in most persons. The right hemisphere plays an important role in visual-spatial-temporal cognitive processing. It is also implicated in discourse semantic processing (Tanner, 2007). According to Gazzaniga, Ivry, and Mangun (1998), the right hemisphere displays superiority in facial recognition and attentional monitoring. Davis (2007) notes that patients with right hemisphere lesions may have anosognosia, the lack of awareness or recognition of disease or disability. The *longitudinal fissure* divides the two hemispheres.

> Each hemisphere consists of an outer layer of cerebral cortex, an intermediate mass of white matter fibers, and an inner mass of gray matter fibers called basal ganglia. Although the brain hemispheres appear identical, the dominant hemisphere is slightly heavier and larger.

The cortex is where most higher level cognitive and intellectual functioning occurs. As can be seen in Figure 1.1, the cerebral cortex is a convoluted structure with ridges or convolutions (gyri) and valleys or depressions (sulci). "If the wrinkled cortex is straightened out to form a flat sheet, we would discover that about two thirds of its surface is hidden in its recesses" (Kent, 1997, p. 243). A major ridge of the cerebral cortex is the *precentral gyrus* also known as the primary motor strip. Major valleys include the *lateral* and *central sulci*. The lateral sulcus is also known as the *Fissure of Sylvius* and the central sulcus is also known as the *Fissure of Rolando*. The approximate boundaries of Broca and Wernicke's areas are shown in Figure 1.1. Broca's area is important for expressive speech and language, and Wernicke's area is its receptive counterpart.

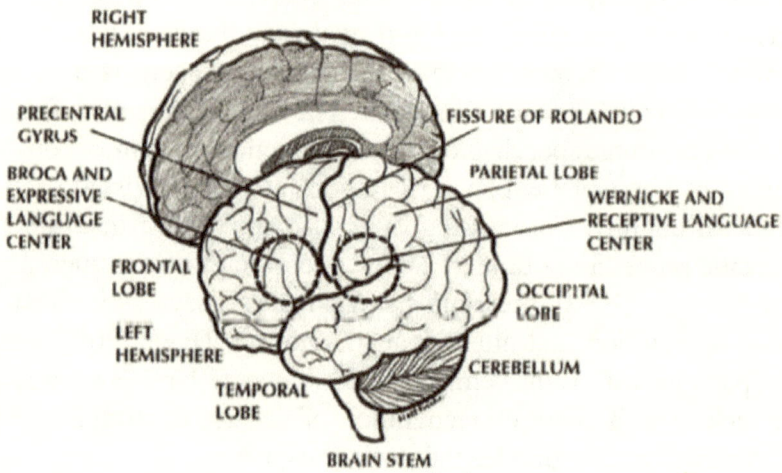

Figure 1.1: Important landmarks of the human brain

> The cerebral cortex is the site of higher mental functions.

Lobes of the Brain

There are four lobes of the brain: *frontal, parietal, temporal,* and *occipital.* The names for the lobes of the brain are based on the bones of the skull under which they are located. The lobes do not operate as independent units although generalities can be drawn about the cognitive, motor, and sensory functioning associated with them.

The frontal lobe is the largest lobe of the brain. The frontal lobe is important to higher level thought processes. Broca's area and the motor cortex are located in the frontal lobe. The central sulcus separates the frontal lobe from the parietal lobe. The parietal lobe is associated with conscious interpretation of tactile information and other functions such as visuospatial processing. It is posterior to the central sulcus and superior to the lateral sulcus. The lateral sulcus separates the temporal and frontal lobes. The temporal lobe is associated with interpretation of auditory input and contains Heschl's Gyrus which is an important site for auditory reception. The occipital lobe is at the posterior region of the brain and is not well-defined. The primary visual cortex is in the occipital lobe.

The Cerebellum

The *cerebellum,* "little brain," is located at the behind and below the cerebral hemispheres. It contains as much as half the total neurons in the central nervous system and has a cortex made up of narrow leaflike folia resembling the pages of a book (Kent, 1997). It has two hemispheres and is connected to the brainstem by the inferior, middle and superior cerebellar peduncies. The cerebellum does not initiate motor activities, but serves as a coordinator. "The functions of the cerebellum are not under voluntary control. In other words, we are not directly aware of the functions of the cerebellum, nor do we voluntarily modify cerebellar functions to any great extent" (Zemlin, 1998, p. 354). It is sometimes called "the great modulator" of muscular movement.

> The cerebellum is connected to the brainstem by three large fiber systems: the inferior, middle, and superior cerebellar peduncles.

Lying below the grey cortex is the subcortical white matter; it is white because a fatty *myelin sheath* covers the axons. The white matter consists of afferent and efferent projection nerve fibers that communicate between other areas of the nervous system. They converge at the *thalami* and *internal capsules* of each hemisphere and descend through the *midbrain, pons,* and *medulla.* The *basal ganglia* are masses of gray matter deep within the cerebrum and there are various ways of categorizing the structures.

The Brainstem

The *brainstem* is an upward extension of the spinal cord and consists of three primary structures: *midbrain, pons,* and *medulla.* Although some authorities list the thalamus as part of the brainstem, it will be dealt with separately. According to Freed (2002, p. 58), the brainstem is important in three ways: "First it acts as a passageway for the descending and ascending neural tracts that travel between the cerebrum and spinal cord. Second, it controls certain integrative and reflexive actions, such as respiration, consciousness, and some parts of the cardiovascular functions. Third, it contains the places where the cranial nerves project out from the CNS, which is probably most important with regard to the motor speech system."

The midbrain contains all of the ascending and many descending systems of the lower brainstem and spinal cord. It also contains the *substaintia nigra* which is important to motor control and the production of dopamine. The pons is a round structure which, in part, relays sensory information between the cerebrum and the cerebellum. The medulla oblongata appears as an expanded section of the spinal cord.

The Thalamus

The *thalamus* is an integrator of sensory information. It is the most central nucleus in the cerebrum with connections to motor, sensory, and association areas of the cortex (Davis, 2007). It is dual lobed and at the top of the brainstem behind the basal ganglia and consists of grey matter. It is sometimes called the "gatekeeper" of information coming from the senses, excluding olfaction, to conscious perception. The hypothalamus lies beneath the thalamus and is important for regulating certain metabolic processes.

Cranial Nerves

Cranial nerves connect the central nervous system to the head and neck (cranial nerve X, the vagus nerve, also connects the central nervous system to the abdomen and thorax). The 12 cranial nerves are numbered from *rostral* (head) to *caudal* (tail). Below are the numbered cranial nerves, their names, sensory and/or motor functioning, and their role in communication where appropriate (Culbertson, Cotton, and Tanner, 2006; Duffy, 2005; Zemlin, 1998).

Cranial Nerve I (Olfactory): This sensory nerve detects chemical changes in the environment and conveys the signal to the cerebral hemispheres to be interpreted as smell. The sense of smell can affect communication ambience.

Cranial Nerve II (Optic): End organs in the retina of the eye generate action potentials that are conveyed to the thalamus by the optic nerve. The impulses are interpreted as vision or stimulate involuntary reactions in the eyes. In communication, the sense of vision is involved in comprehending bodily gestures, reading, writing, and interpreting facial expressions.

Cranial Nerve III (Oculomotor): This motor nerve, originating in the midbrain, reacts to input from the optic nerve and from the voluntary eye field of the cerebral cortex to activate and coordinate most of the extrinsic and all of the intrinsic muscle movements of the eye including focusing and pupil dilation.

Cranial Nerve IV (Trochlear): This motor nerve originates in the midbrain and causes the eye to look out and down, and thus assisting visual tracking during reading.

Cranial Nerve V (Trigeminal): Originating in the pons, this motor and sensory nerve conveys motor impulses for the jaw and sensation from the face, mouth, tongue, and jaw. For speech purposes, it is important for elevation of the mandible during articulation.

Cranial Nerve VI (Abducens): This motor and sensory nerve originates in the pons and pulls the eyeball to the side and out during visual tracking.

Cranial Nerve VII (Facial): Originating in the pons, this motor and sensory nerve is involved in facial movements and conveys the sense of taste from the anterior two-thirds of the tongue.

Cranial Nerve VIII (Vestibulocochlear): Also known as the auditory-vestibular cranial nerve, it originates in the pons and medulla. It is the sensory nerve for hearing and balance.

Cranial Nerve IX (Glossopharyngeal). The glossopharyngeal nerve originates in the medulla and is both sensory and motor. It conveys taste and touch sensations from the oropharynx to the central nervous system and is involved in pharyngeal movement (stylopharyngeus).

Cranial Nerve X (Vagus). Originating in the medulla, this motor and sensory nerve supplies smooth muscle motor function to the pharynx, thorax, and some abdominal muscles. Afferent functions of the vagus nerve include conscious and unconscious somesthesis of the pharynx and thorax. It also innervates the larynx.

Cranial Nerve XI (Accessory). The accessory cranial nerve, a motor nerve originating in the medulla and spinal cord, accompanies the vagus nerve to supply voluntary innervation to the intrinsic laryngeal muscles, pharyngeal constrictors and palatal elevators.

Cranial Nerve XII (Hypoglossal). Originating in the medulla, this motor nerve is the final common pathway for motor innervation to the intrinsic and most of the extrinsic tongue muscles.

Table 1.1 shows the cranial nerves, whether they are motor, sensory, or both, and their general function.

Table 1.1: Cranial Nerves and General Functions

I	Olfactory	Sensory	Smell
II	Optic	Sensory	Vision
III	Oculomotor	Motor	Eye movements
IV	Trochlear	Motor	Eye movements
V	Trigeminal	Motor and Sensory	Jaw movements and sensation to the face, jaw, and mouth
VI	Abducens	Motor	Eye movements
VII	Facial	Motor and Sensory	Facial movements and taste
VIII	Vestibulocochlear	Sensory	Balance and hearing
IX	Glossopharyngeal	Motor and Sensory	Pharyngeal movements, tongue sensation, and taste
X	Vagus	Motor and Sensory	Motor to pharyngeal, palatal, laryngeal, and some abdominal muscles, pharyngeal sensation
XI	Accessory	Motor	Shoulder, neck, and laryngeal movements
XII	Hypoglossal	Motor	Tongue movements

Some anatomists consider the olfactory and optic nerves part of the central nervous system.

Spinal Nerves

The 31 spinal nerves are divided into five regions: *cervical, thoracic, lumbar, sacral,* and *coccygeal.* The most important speech function of the spinal nerves is for respiratory support. The *diaphragm* is innervated by the *phrenic nerves* which receive fibers from the cervical plexus. Motor innervation of the upper extremities is provided through the nerves of the brachial plexus, thus playing an important role in writing and gestures.

> The spinal cord is the caudal extension of the brainstem and its functions are said to be segmental.

Neurons

While neurons come in different sizes and shapes, they all contain a *cell body, axon,* and *dendrites.* Neurons have one axon and the diameter of the axon varies with its length (Duffy, 2005). Dendrites are shorter, have many branches, and gather information from other neurons. "The duties of a dendrite are always to conduct impulses toward the cell body, while the duties of axons are to conduct impulses away from the cell body" (Zemlin, 1998, p. 382). Many long axons have a myelin sheath, a fatty substance which accelerates propagation of action potentials. The synapse is where communication between neurons, glands, and muscles occur and is a function of *neurotransmitters.* Neurotransmitters are chemical messengers that enter a synapse and facilitate the propagation of action potentials from one neuron to another. Love and Webb (1996, pp. 68-69) succinctly describes the process:

> For a neural impulse to be generated, the membrane of a neuron must open for a brief time to allow positively charged sodium ions to flow into the cell, which is normally negatively charged. This flow of ions will effect a change in polarization (or a depolarization) if continued and the cell will become positively charged. The positive charge causes

an action potential or electrical charge to be emitted. This action potential is essentially the neural impulse. The action potential travels down the axon until it reaches the area of synapse (literally, "union") with another neuron, a muscle or a gland. The area on this axon is called the presynaptic terminal of the membrane. The action potential causes a release of a substance called a neurotransmitter into the postsynaptic terminal of the membrane of the other neuron. At this point another action potential may be effected or other types of potentials may occur.

Blood Supply to the Brain

The heart propels blood through the cardiovascular system. Blood flows from the heart through arteries and returns through veins. During its flow, blood exchanges gases in the lungs, is filtered in the liver and kidneys, and receives nutrients in the digestive system. According to Davis (2007), the blood supply to the brain has three structural levels: arteries in the neck, interconnecting arteries in the base of the brain, and cerebral arteries on the surface of the cortex.

> Blood consists of formed elements included red blood cells (erythrocytes), several types of white blood cells (leukocytes), and platelets (thrombocytes).

The *internal carotid* arteries and the *vertebral* arteries transport blood in the neck. The vertebral arteries join to become the basilar artery which supplies blood to the cerebellum and brainstem. The cerebral arteries begin in the *Circle of Willis* at the base of the brain. "This polygon of small arteries is one collateral system in which some compensation may occur for occlusion in a carotid artery below" (Davis, 2007, p. 20). The anterior cerebral artery primarily serves the medial frontal and parietal lobes. The posterior cerebral artery primarily serves the posterior aspects of the occipital lobe. The middle cerebral artery serves the major speech and language centers of the brain.

Etiology of Neurogenic Communication Disorders

Although there are literally hundreds of causal agents and etiological factors in neurogenic communication disorders, most can be included in the following categories: *strokes, cancer and other diseases,* and *traumatic brain injury.*

Stroke

Strokes are the third-leading cause of death in the United States and are the most common cause of aphasia, apraxia of speech, and several dysarthrias. Strokes deprive the brain of blood, and when it is deprived to the brain for longer than about two minutes, neural tissue dies. There are two categories of vascular disturbances resulting in neurogenic communication disorders: *occlusive* and *hemorrhagic.*

An occlusive vascular accident is the result of the blockage of an artery. A blood clot or other obstruction can cause the blockage. It can also be caused by gradual decrease in the opening of blood vessels. When the blockage originates in the brain, it is called a cerebral thrombosis. "Most strokes are a thrombosis, which occurs from accumulation of atherosclerotic platelet and fatty plaque on the vessel wall at the site of occlusion" (Davis, 2007, p. 20). A cerebral embolus is a blockage originating elsewhere in the body and eventually lodging in the brain. Two or more emboli are called a *shower of emboli.* How much brain damage that occurs is dependent upon the completeness of the blockage and the size of the area of the brain deprived of blood. When a small area of the brain is deprived of blood, there is generally less damage to communicative functions than if the damaged area were large. However, some small focalized areas of brain damage may cause major neurogenic communication disorders.

A *transient ischemic attack* (TIA) is sometimes referred to as a ministroke. It is a temporary disruption of blood flow in the brain and often foretells an impending stroke. During a transient ischemic attack, the patient may have neurogenic communication disorders typical of a stroke, which remit after the TIA is over. A *stroke-in-evolution* is an ongoing disruption in blood flow to the brain.

A hemorrhagic stroke is caused by a blowout of a blood vessel and is usually associated with high blood pressure. A ruptured aneurysm causes some hemorrhages. An aneurysm is a weakening of the arterial wall and a ballooning of an artery. When a blood vessel hemorrhages, the area served by the vessel is deprived of blood and there is spilling of it elsewhere often causing increased pressure in the brain and restricting blood flow. The accumulated blood is called a *hematoma* and may have to be evacuated by a neurosurgeon.

Cancer and Other Diseases

A tumor is also called a *neoplasm* and it may be *benign* or *malignant*. Benign tumors are space-occupying and can cause neurogenic communication disorders. Malignant neoplasms grow uncontrolled and can metastasize or spread to other parts of the body. The types of neurogenic communication disorder caused by tumors depend on their severity and where in the neurological system they occur. Malignant cerebral neoplasms, brain tumors, can cause aphasia and other neurogenic communication disorders depending on the brain tissue affected and the reduced blood circulation caused by increased cranial pressure. Surgeries and other treatments for cancer may also damage tissue and cause neurogenic communication disorders.

Other diseases that can cause neurogenic communication disorders include those that affect neuromuscular functioning, motor speech programming and execution, and language functions. For example, progressive degenerative diseases such as *amyotrophic lateral sclerosis, muscular dystrophy,* and *multiple sclerosis* impair neuromuscular functioning. *Parkinson's disease,* caused by the deficiency of the neurotransmitter dopamine, disrupts neuromuscular functioning. *Alzheimer's* and other dementia causing diseases can affect motor speech programming and execution. Any disease affecting cognition can disrupt or destroy normal expressive and receptive language functions.

Traumatic Brain Injury

There are two types of head injuries: *closed* and *open*. A closed head injury is caused by a blunt force trauma to the head resulting in acceleration and deceleration of the brain. When this occurs, axons within the brain are torn. In an open head injury, a projectile or missile penetrates the skull and brain. Common projectiles include bullets fired from guns and shrapnel. Both open and closed head traumas can cause focalized and diffuse brain injuries and hemorrhages. Traumatic brain injury can minimally or completely disrupt language, motor speech programming and execution, and neuromuscular functioning. The site, extent, and nature of the traumatic brain injury determine the symptoms presented by the patient. Because traumatic brain injuries are so variable, there are three diagnostic factors related to the etiology of neurogenic communication disorders (Tanner, 2006a, 2003).

> There are about 500,000 traumatic brain injury hospitalizations each year in the United States (Ylvisaker, Szekeres, and Feeney, 2001).

First, a small percentage of traumatic brain injured persons primarily have focalized damage to the major speech and language centers of the brain. Because there is focalized damage, they have neurogenic communication disorders typically seen in many stroke patients. Second, some patients have traumatically induced brain and/or central nervous system damage, but the major speech and language centers are spared. Although these patients may have problems communicating, the fabric of language and the motor speech functions remain intact. These patients primarily present with arousal, orientation, behavior, and judgment disorders, and amnesia. Third, traumatic brain injured patients, particularly those with severe injuries, often have aphasia, apraxia of speech, and the dysarthrias compounded by arousal, orientation, behavior, and judgment disorders, and amnesia.

The Brain-Mind Leap

An issue that has challenged neuroscientists, theologians, and philosophers for centuries is the so-called *brain-mind leap*. The brain-mind leap is the scientific and philosophical process of projecting the neurological activity in the brain and nervous system to what occurs in a person's mind. At the brain level, consciousness, thought, and speech and language are electrochemical impulses traveling along nerve axons to synaptic junctions. As discussed previously, neurological impulses are actions of nerve fibers and electrical charges traveling from neuron to neuron and involving several chemical reactions at the synaptic level. The neuron propagates ionic changes, action potentials, which travel from dendrites to axons. All changes in consciousness, thought, and speech and language are the result of changes in brain chemistry and new neuronal connections. The scientific, religious, and philosophical issues in the brain-mind leap are how these chemical and neuronal activities in a person's brain become consciousness, thought, and speech and language.

> According to Davis (2007), aphasiology was born with a neurological orientation more than one hundred years ago, whereas a scientific approach to the mind emerged only since the 1970s.

No better example exists of the difficulties and challenges involved in the brain-mind leap than in language functioning, and particularly abstract semantics.

The magnitude of the brain-mind leap can be demonstrated by addressing semantic representations in the brain. Neurologically, the meaning of the word "truthfulness," for example, can be found in the atomic particles in neurons, and the chemical interactions of neurotransmitters at their synaptic junctions. The meaning of the word "truthfulness" is likely a composite of these changes to cellular chemistry and continuous action potentials in thousands of neurons and their dendrite-to-axon connections. These electrochemical reactions somehow create the continuous imagery and semantic associations necessary to sense the meaning of the word and to use it expressively. Interestingly, the neuronal impulses, their action potentials, and cellular chemical stores have continuity. They are consistent from one semantic retrieval to another, yet the meaning of the word evolves with life experience. Through this ongoing continuous nervous energy and chemical changes at the cellular level, a person is conscious of the meaning of "truthfulness," and in fact, the semantics of the word becomes part of his or her consciousness (Tanner, 2006b, pp. 162-163).

According to Davis (2007, p. 9), "The brain and the mind are not usually treated as alternative versions of the truth."

Language and the Localization Movement

Integrally tied to the brain-mind leap in neurogenic communication disorders is the *localization* movement. It formally began in 1865 when Pierre Paul Broca discovered that expressive speech and language functions occur in the frontal lobe of the left hemisphere in most persons. He announced this localization of specific speech and language functions in the brain with the now-famous statement: "We speak with the left hemisphere."

No one would argue that speech and language functioning is localized to the brain and nervous system in humans. About 4000 years ago, the ancient Egyptians tied brain damage to speechlessness. Early Greek and Roman philosophers understood that speech and language are inherently related to brain and nervous system functioning. The central question that evolved over time was the role of language in thought. Specifically with regard to neurogenic communication disorders, the question arose about thought processes in persons deprived of language, i.e., patients with global aphasia. Currently, there are two schools of thought about language, thought, and aphasia: *associationists* and *cognitivists*.

> Henry Head was an early critic of the brain localization movement and sarcastically referred to localizationists as "diagram makers."

Associationists believe that patients with aphasia have disturbances in labeling events, objects, and ideas. Because of damage to the language centers of the brain, aphasic patients simply have problems retrieving words to express their unimpaired thought processes. Associationists believe that intelligence remains essentially intact in patients deprived of language; intelligence is located outside the major language centers of the brain. Cognitivists challenge the idea that language is simply a labeling system in adults. According to the cognitive school of thought, because language and thought are integrally tied throughout the brain, aphasic patients are cognitively impaired. The impairment is most apparent in verbal thought processes, especially abstract language, but the cognitive impairments also transcend to nonverbal processes such as categorization and object matching-to-sample tasks.

Today, neuroscientists and aphasiologists search for *brain modules*. Modules are areas of the brain devoted to specific processing activities or function (Owens, Metz, and Haas, 2000). A strict localizationist philosophy of brain functioning and the associationist school of thought with regard to language processing is difficult to support because the brain operates holistically. No single part of the brain functions completely independent from other areas. For example, Ackermann (2007) using brain imaging of normal speakers repeating syllables found the *supplemental motor area, bilateral sensorimotor cortex, bilateral basal ganglia, left anterior insula,* both *cerebellar hemispheres,* and *the left inferior frontal gyrus* (Broca's area) are active in this simple motor speech task. He notes that damage to these structures may give rise to dysarthria (See Chapter 6), apraxia of speech (See Chapter 5) or impaired speech initiation mechanisms. This holistic brain activity is particularly true with regard to language processing; language involves global sensation, perception, and association and it virtually engages the brain and nervous system as a whole. This is not to say that modules do not exist that are important for certain language functions, especially motor and sensory processing. However, attempting to pinpoint a focalized mass of brain cells or a neuronal tract completely responsible for interpreting a proverb or understanding a poem is absurd (Tanner, 2007).

Overview of the Psychology of Neurogenic Communication Disorders

Over the past 30 years, there have been more than one hundred studies conducted of the efficacy of therapy for patients with neurogenic communication disorders. While most research shows that therapies for neurogenic communication disorders are effective and worthwhile for speech and language recovery, they also suggest that they are valuable psychologically. For both patients and family members, the support, direction, and guidance provided by clinicians are important, if not necessary, to optimal recovery. This places a premium on clinicians being aware of the multiple psychological factors associated with neurogenic communication disorders. Unfortunately, this is a neglected academic and clinical subject in most college and university training programs in communication sciences and disorders. For example, while clinicians must learn much about the neurology of communication disorders, of which they can do nothing to change for the patient, the psychology of these disorders is addressed minimally or neglected altogether. In addition, most textbooks on neurogenic communication disorders relegate the psychological aspects of these disorders to the end of the book almost as an incidental afterthought, if the authors deal with them at all. Nearly a half century ago, Schuell, Jenkins, and Jimenez-Pabon (1964, p. 315) in their classic text, *Aphasia in Adults*, addressed the importance of the psychology of neurogenic communication disorders:

> To say a clinician must be aware of psychological problems in aphasia is to say he must be aware that he is dealing with people. Sometimes we are so intimidated by labels, such as emotional lability, catastrophic reactions, anxiety, depression, euphoria, etc., that we forget this first

principle. We talk trade jargon with glibness that betrays our dearth of insights. We talk as though aphasic patients were different from everyone else, and we had to have a different set of rules for dealing with them.

According to Tetnowski (2003, p. x): "Psychological issues can have an impact on otherwise clear, understandable diagnoses. If we are to treat the whole person, we must understand the importance of psychological factors surrounding neurogenic communication disorders."

John Hughlings Jackson (1835-1911), considered by many to be the father of British neurology, was the first systematically to study aphasia and related disorders from a psychological perspective. While Sigmund Freud also addressed aphasia and the unconscious mind, John Hughlings Jackson proposed a unitary, psychological approach to brain functioning and extended it to the study of aphasia (Benson and Ardila, 1996). According to Sies (1974), Jackson addressed the idea of *inner speech* and applied it to neurogenic communication disorders. Jackson did not artificially separate the aphasia patient's psyche from his or her cognition, speech and language processes, and his or her intent during communication. Since Jackson's groundbreaking work on the psychology of neurogenic communication disorders, three issues have evolved that challenge current scientists and clinicians: *psycho-organic factors, loss of verbal defense mechanisms,* and the *grief response* (Tanner, 2009; Tanner, 2003).

The first issue in the psychology of neurogenic communication disorders concerns brain and nervous system damage per se. It has long been known that certain psychological, emotional, and behavioral reactions occur because of brain and nervous system damage. These psychological, emotional, and behavioral reactions range from excessive crying to euphoria. Scientists and clinicians are currently investigating the relationships of these psychological, emotional, and behavioral reactions to the nature and extent of the neurological damage.

The second issue currently being addressed in neurogenic communication disorders concerns *psychological defenses* and *coping styles*. All persons use defense mechanisms and coping styles to deal with anxiety and stress. Some defense mechanisms and coping styles are mature, adaptive, and lead to mental health while others are immature, radical, and desperate attempts to deal with unpleasantness. Patients with neurogenic communication disorders employ them with differing degrees of success as a consequence of their neurogenic communication disorders. Of particular interest is how the loss of language seen in aphasic persons affects these defense mechanisms and coping styles. Some defense mechanisms and coping styles are nonverbal, such as denial, while others are verbal, such as rationalization. Aphasic patients are deprived of many verbal defense mechanisms due to their loss of language.

The third psychological issue concerns how patients cope with *unwanted change*. Patients with neurogenic communication disorders often experience permanent separation from abilities, loved ones, and valued objects. These patients, like all persons, can be expected to grieve over those losses and to pass through predictable stages of accepting unwanted changes. While there is individual variability in these grieving stages, and special issues associated with impaired or lost abilities to communicate, most patients with neurogenic communication disorders feel a deep sense of loss and grieve over the loss of communication with loved ones, physical abilities, and valued objects. Lyon and Shadden (2001) and Code, Hemsley, and Herrmann (1999) note that the grief model can explain some of the psychosocial and emotional reactions seen in aphasia.

While there is overlap in the above three aspects of the psychology of neurogenic communication disorders, each of them, more or less, play a role in the patient's psychology and adjustment to the disability. Some patients are more psychologically affected by the brain and nervous system damage. Other patients experience more grief reactions, and still others, such as global aphasics, have reduced abilities to cope due to the loss of verbal psychological defenses and coping styles. Many neurogenic communication disorders are major life-altering events and understanding the patient's psychology is fundamental to helping him or her return to a meaningful and fulfilling quality of life.

> Psychologically, neurogenic communication disorders are double-edged swords. Serious medical conditions often cause them, bringing on many adjustment challenges, and they can sever communication between the patient and his or her loved ones.

Neurogenic Communication Disorders and Quality of Life

Although *quality of life* is an important topic when discussing the human life experience, it is rarely defined. When discussing quality of life, most people simply assume there is a general consensus about what it is for all people, at all ages, and under all circumstances. What is most important, there is a general belief that what is a good or poor quality of life for one person will be the same for another. In fact, the factors that contribute or detract from quality of life are highly variable. One person's idea of a good quality of life may be viewed as an impoverished existence by another.

Lawton (1991) defines quality of life as having four critical domains which interact with each other: *psychological well-being, perceived quality of life, behavioral competence,* and *objective environment.* With regard to individuals with neurogenic communication disorders, an all-encompassing fourth dimension, communication competence, is a necessary component to understanding quality of life issues in persons with significantly reduced abilities to communicate.

Psychological Well-Being

A person must be free of mental illness to experience a good quality of life. No one would argue that having a good quality of life is impossible for a person who is in the grips of a deep depression or suffering the anxiety of frequent panic attacks. However, a sense of psychological well-being is more than being free of mental illness. It is also having a reason to live, optimism about life in general, spiritual meaningfulness, and social contacts with whom to share life's journey. Underlying the sense of well-being are brain chemicals, particularly serotonin and dopamine, when in proper balance, are biological agents contributing to a positive emotional state.

The opposite of a sense of psychological well-being is depression. To some neuroscientists and localizationist, non-grieving depression is an imbalance of chemicals in the brain. To some mental health authorities, people get depressed because they do not produce "feel good" chemicals in adequate amounts or they are eliminated too quickly from the body. The result is having an inadequate level of these chemicals thus causing various degrees of depression. The medical treatment for depression is the administration of *antidepressants*. The current generation of antidepressants result in higher levels of these mood enhancing chemicals in the patient's brain and are remarkably free of serious side-effects in adults. In neurogenic communication disorders, the depression seen in many patients is caused by a chemical imbalance resulting from damage to specific areas of the brain and nervous system.

A social and psychotherapeutic explanation for depression is that it is primarily stress-induced. It is common for a person to suffer from high levels of stress preceding or during the onset of the depression. The stress can be positive or negative. For example, loss of a job is negatively stressful while being promoted to a new one can be positively stressful. The relationship between stress and depression is highly variable and what one person finds stressful another may not. When under chronic stress, some persons feel depressed, hopeless, and helpless. Through counseling and psychotherapy, depressed persons learn to cope with stress and depression.

While it may seem that the above chemical and stress explanations for a sense of psychological well-being are unrelated, they may be integrally tied to each other. An individual's nonadaptive way of dealing with stress may cause a reduction in serotonin and other mood enhancing brain chemicals. In effect, stress and a person's inability to properly deal with it may cause brain chemistry to go awry. Because of this brain-mind relationship, most treatments of depression involve counseling and psychotherapy and the administration of antidepressants if necessary.

Communication competence is necessary for a sense of psychological well-being. Most persons need to be able to communicate with others about important aspects of their lives and the emotions associated with life changes. In addition, counseling and psychotherapy are "talking cures" for depression and other psychological disorders. For individuals with neurogenic communication disorders, their significant communication disorders can create barriers to overcoming depression and a reduced sense of psychological well-being.

Perceived Quality of Life

As reported above, perceived quality of life is a subjective estimate and differs from one person to the next. If one perceives that he or she is experiencing a good quality of life, this belief actually contributes to it. Conversely, if a person feels that his or her life is impoverished, then this perception contributes to a poor quality of life. Other than health, there are few objective events or situations that are universally perceived to contribute to quality of life. Even wealth is not necessarily associated with a high quality of living. Perception of one's quality of life is fundamentally tied to a person's *self-esteem.*

Self-esteem is a positive belief and feeling about one's self. According to Stuart (2001), a person's self-esteem is derived from perceptions of self and the judgments of others. Joseph Wepman (1962), an early aphasiologist, observed that in all instances of brain damage, there is some reduction in the patient's self-esteem. For persons with neurogenic communication disorders, their previous beliefs and attitudes about disabled persons will affect their self-esteem and quality of life. Brumfitt (1996) observes that an aphasic patient's identity must change based on the new disability.

Sarno (1991) defines aphasia as a "disorder of person" rather than a "disorder of language" recognizing the major effects of this neurogenic communication disorder on the patient's personality. Jon Eisenson (1984, p. 87) addressed ego involvement and aphasia: "We would consider it surprising if an individual who has incurred a cerebral insult and associated aphasic disturbances did not undergo consequent changes in personality." Eisenson notes that those patients who adjust to the brain damage go on to make good recoveries. Regaining self-esteem, even with the knowledge that one has sustained brain damage and disabilities, shows a positive reorganization of the ego and self-concept.

Perceived quality of life is affected by the way patients adapt to *chronic illness*. According to LaPointe (1997), successful adaptation to chronic illness involves going from uncertainty to regaining wellness through taking charge, setting goals, seeking closure, and attaining mastery over the illness. The patient's communication competence is important to successful adaptation to disabilities and regaining a positive perceived quality of life. Positive perceptions of the patient's neurogenic communication disorder can be facilitated by the rehabilitation team working together on psychiatric factors (Frank, 1998).

Behavioral Competence

Behavioral competence is the patient's ability to exercise control over his or her environment. People who can exert control over their lives are less likely to suffer depression and the hopelessness and helplessness that often accompanies it. For patients with neurogenic communication disorders, the physical disabilities that often accompany these disorders can limit behavioral competence. Hemiparalysis which often co-occurs with many neurogenic communication disorders is a significant deterrent to behavior competence.

Hemiparalysis affects behavioral competence particularly with regard to activities of daily living. Hemiparalysis can disrupt or eliminate the patient's ability to walk, dress, eat, groom, and independently go to the bathroom. These limitations dramatically affect the patient's quality of life. Regaining wellness and attaining mastery over the disabilities is due, in no small part, to the success of occupational, vocational, and physical therapies in addressing the hemiparalysis.

Perhaps the most significant behavioral competence limitations are neurogenic communication disorders that render patients functionally unable to communicate. Communication is the primary way people exercise control over their environments. Whether it is a business executive directing the course of his or her corporation through communication with subordinates, or a husband and wife negotiating the responsibilities of child care, communication is indispensable to exercising control of one's affairs. Nonfunctional communication abilities deprived patients with even a modicum of control over their environments. To show the importance of functional communication on quality of life, in a study addressing laryngeal cancer, MacNeil, Weischselbaum, and Parker (1981) found that most of the subjects were willing to trade off life expectancy to retain the ability to speak. For patients with neurogenic communication disorders, achieving any degree of functional speech and language or utilizing alternative communication systems are essential to regaining a good quality of life.

> Quality of life, standard of living, and happiness are terms often used interchangeably.

Objective Environment

Some patients with neurogenic communication disorders are institutionalized. The quality of long-term rehabilitation centers, nursing homes, and other extended care facilities varies greatly and can significantly affect a patient's quality of life. Some facilities provide optimal long-term services to disabled persons that contribute to high quality living. The food is healthy and patients receive a balanced diet. There are recreational activities, reading rooms, media centers, solariums, clubs, sports, and exercise programs. The medical, nursing, and rehabilitation programs in these facilities are of the highest quality. Unfortunately, there are other facilities that do not provide the necessary objective environment for quality living.

The objective environment for patients who return home also varies greatly. Some objective home environments are loving, healthy, stimulating, and provide more than the essentials to achieving a high quality of life for the patient. Many patients are positively reintegrated into the family roles and responsibilities reflecting their abilities to communicate. As with long-term care institutions, there are also patients who return to a home where the objective environment is far less than optimal and detracts from quality living.

Two political and technological factors have improved the objective environments for disabled persons. First, the 1990 *Americans with Disabilities Act* has open many doors for persons with neurogenic communication disorders. This congressional act, and other legislation, have made aspects of society more accessible to the disabled. No longer is it legal to discriminate against disabled persons in employment, housing, education, transportation, recreation, voting, and access to public services. Second, major advances in *technology* have also improved disabled persons' objective environment. Communication boards, speech synthesizers, voice recognition devices, scanning instruments, digital hearing aids, personal computers, and cochlear implants have increased social and vocational opportunities for millions of disabled persons. Together, legislation benefitting the disabled population and technological advances have greatly improved the social inclusion of the disabled and ultimately their quality of lives.

Chapter Summary

Neurogenic communication disorders involve damage to the brain and nervous system and are caused by strokes, cancer and other diseases, and traumatic brain injuries. While neurogenic communication disorders are interesting to study and transcend several academic and clinical disciplines, they can be devastating to persons suffering from them. Broadly defined, neurogenic communication disorders include aphasia, apraxia of speech, agnosia, the language of confusion, and the dysarthrias. An important and challenging issue to understanding neurogenic communication disorders is the brain-mind leap. The psychology of neurogenic communication disorders includes addressing psycho-organic factors, loss of verbal defense mechanisms and coping styles, and the patient's reactions to loss. An important issue in neurogenic communication disorders is the effects of the disabilities on the patient's quality of life.

Study and Discussion Questions

1. List and define the primary neurogenic communication disorders.
2. What disciplines study and treat neurogenic communication disorders?
3. Describe the brain hemispheres.
4. List and describe the lobes of the brain.
5. List the cranial nerves and describe their functions with regard to communication.
6. How does a neuron work?
7. Describe the blood supply to the brain.
8. List and describe the etiological factors associated with neurogenic communication disorders.
9. What is the brain-mind leap and how does it relate to the localization movement?
10. Discuss the psychology of neurogenic communication disorders and relate it to quality of life.

References

Ackermann, H. (2007, September). Glimpses into the speaking brain: Imaging techniques provide new insight into speech motor control. *The ASHA Leader*, Vol. 12, No. 12: 10-13.

Benson, D. and Ardila, A. (1996). *Aphasia*. New York: Oxford University Press.

Brumfitt, S. (1996). Losing your sense of self: What aphasia can do. In *Forums in clinical aphasiology*, C. Code, (Ed). London: Whurr Publishers.

Code, C., Hemsley, G., and Herrmann, M. (1999). The emotional impact of aphasia. *Seminars in speech and language*, 20(1): 19-31.

Culbertson, W. R., Cotton, S.S., and Tanner, D.C. (2006). *Anatomy and physiology study guide for speech and hearing.* San Diego: Plural Publishing.

Davis, G.A. (2007). *Aphasiology: Disorders and clinical practice* (2nd ed.) Boston: Pearson, Allyn and Bacon.

Duffy, J.R. (2005). *Motor speech disorders: Substrates, differential diagnosis, and management* (2nd ed.). St. Louis: Mosby.

Eisenson, J. (1984). *Adult aphasia*, (2nd ed.). Englewood Cliffs, NJ: Prentice-Hall.

Frank, C. (1998). Overview of psychiatric disease for the speech-language practitioner. In *Medical speech-language pathology: A practitioner's guide.* A. Johnson and B. Jacobson (Eds). New York: Thieme.

Freed, D.B. (2002). *Motor speech disorders: Diagnosis and treatment.* San Diego: Plural Publishing.

Gazzaniga, M.., Ivry, R., and Mangun, G. (1998). *Cognitive neuroscience: The biology of the mind.* New York: W.W. Norton and Company.

Kent, R. D. (1997). *The speech sciences.* San Diego: Singular Publishing Group.

Kirshner, H. (1995). Cerebral cortex: Higher mental functions. In S. Bhatnagar and O. Andy (Eds). *Neuroscience for the study of communicative disorders.* Baltimore: Williams & Wilkins.

LaPointe, L. (1997). Adaptation, accommodation, aristos. In *Aphasia and related neurogenic language disorders* (2nd ed.). L. LaPointe (Ed). New York: Thieme.

Lawton, M. (1991). A multidimensional view of quality of life in frail elders. In *The concept and measurement of quality of life in frail elders*. J. Birren (Ed). San Diego: Academic Press.

Love, R. J. And Webb, W.G. (1996). *Neurology for the speech-language pathologist* (3rd ed.). Boston: Butterworth-Heinemann.

Lyon, J. and Shadden, B. (2001). Treating life consequences of aphasia's chronicity. In *Language intervention in aphasia and related neurogenic communication disorders* (4th ed.). R. Chapey (Ed). Philadelphia: Lippincott Williams and Wilkins.

MacNeil, B., Weischselbaum, R., and Pauker, S. (1981). Tradeoffs between quality and quantity of life in laryngeal cancer. *New England Journal of Medicine,* 305: 983-987.

Owens, R., Metz, D., and Haas, A. (2000). *Introduction to communication disorders.* Boston: Allyn & Bacon.

Ruben, R.J. (2000). Redefining the survival of the fittest: Communication disorders in the 21st century. *Laryngoscope, 110*: 241-245.

Sarno, M. (1991). Treatment of aphasia workshop research and research needs. *Aphasia treatment: Current approaches and research opportunities,* 2, xi-xvi.

Schuell, H., Jenkins, J., and Jimenez-Pabon, E. (1964). *Aphasia in adults.* New York: Harper and Row.

Sies, L. (1974). *Aphasia: Theory and therapy.* Baltimore: University Park Press.

Stuart, G. (1998). Self-concept responses and dissociative disorders. In *Principles and practice of psychiatric nursing (7ᵗʰ ed.)* (pp. 274-298), G. Stuart and M. Laraia (Eds). St. Louis: Mosby

Tanner, D. (2003, Winter). Eclectic perspectives on the psychology of aphasia. *J. Allied Health: 32:256-260.*

Tanner, D. (2009). *The psychology of neurogenic communication disorders: A primer for health care professionals.* New York: iUniverse.

Tanner, D. (2006a). *Case studies in communication sciences and disorders.* Upper Saddle River, N.J.: Pearson Merrill Prentice Hall.

Tanner, D. (2006b). *An advanced course in communication sciences and disorders.* San Diego: Plural Publishing.

Tanner, D. (2007). Redefining Wernicke's area: Receptive language and discourse semantics. *J Allied Health, 36:63-66.*

Tetnowski, J.A (2003). Foreword. *The psychology of neurogenic communication disorders: A primer for health care professionals.* Boston: Allyn and Bacon.

Wepman, J. (1962). The language disorders. In *Psychological practices with the physically disabled,* J. Garrett and E. Levine (Eds). New York: Columbia University Press.

Ylvisaker, M., Szekeres, S.F., and Feeney, T. (2001). Communication disorders associated with traumatic brain injury. In R. Chapey (Ed), *Language intervention strategies in aphasia and related neurogenic communication disorders* (4th ed.) (pp. 745-808). Philadelphia: Lippincott Williams & Wilkins.

Zemlin, W.R. (1998). *Speech and hearing science: Anatomy and physiology.* Boston: Allyn and Bacon.

Chapter Two: History of Neurogenic Communication Disorders

> "Those who cannot remember the past are condemned to repeat it."
>
> George Santayana

Chapter Preview: This chapter explores the study and treatment of neurogenic communication disorders. Examined are the ancient Egyptian, Greek, and Roman views of the brain and nervous system, and the effects of neurological damage on the ability to communicate. There is a summary of the study and treatment of neurogenic communication disorders during the middle ages and the enlightenment that occurred during the Renaissance. In this chapter, Pierre Paul Broca and Karl Wernicke's identification of speech and language functions are detailed and there is a historical overview of theories about the brain, nervous system, and neurogenic communication disorders occurring to the present-day.

Why Study the History of Neurogenic Communication Disorders

Our current understanding of the human brain, nervous system, and muscles of the body is the cumulative product of thousands of years of theorizing, philosophizing, and scientific advances. Much of what we now know about the neurosciences is the outcome of studying, not normal brains, nervous systems, and muscles, but the thousands of diseases, disorders, and defects that can wreak havoc on them. And because communication is the highest and most evolved function of which humans are capable, the study of neurogenic communication disorders has and continues to be central to the acquisition of knowledge about the neurosciences. The act of speech communication involves thought, language, motor speech programming, and the five basic motor speech processes: respiration, phonation, articulation, resonance, and prosody. Reading, writing, and mathematics are sophisticated learned cognitive and linguistic functions and the myriad of disorders affecting these high level processes and functions provide valuable insight into their fundamental nature. Neurogenic communication disorders, perhaps more than any other human malady, have directly and indirectly contributed vast amounts of information about the general functioning of the brain, nervous system, and muscles of the body. Sies (1974) notes that few human maladies have generated more confusion, promoted more heated controversy among professional workers, or caused more human suffering than neurogenic communication disorders.

Primitive humans suffered brain and nervous system damage and they attempted to cure disease and disorders through crude surgeries. Archeological records show examples of hominid skulls with fatal cranial damage dating back one million years. Archeologists have discovered holes bored in human skulls, evidently as a cure for disease, dating 10,000 years ago (Bear, Connors, and Paradiso, 1998). These primitive humans, at an instinctual level, understood the importance of the brain and nervous system and practiced rudimentary medical treatments to cure diseases and disorders.

The Ancient Egyptians

About 4000 years ago, the ancient Egyptians systematically studied the brain, nervous system, and neurogenic communication disorders. In an ancient Egyptian surgical text, the first medical textbook, there are 48 case studies beginning with injuries to the head and systematically moving downward in the body. O'Neill (1980) notes that Case 22 was a patient with a "smash to his temple," and for the first time in written history, speechlessness and brain injury were linked, the cerebral convolutions were compared to corrugations on a metallic slag, and the *meninges* likened to a sack. "The Egyptian surgeons believed that loss of speech resulted from 'something entering from the outside,' like 'the breath of an outside god or death,' and that the patient 'was silent in sadness' (Schuell, Jenkins, and Jimenez-Pabon, 1964, p. 11). The ancient Egyptian physicians did not believe the patient's communication disorder was treatable.

"Included in an ancient Egyptian hieroglyphic report was a description of a patient with a head wound: "...one having a wound in his temple, perforating his temporal bone; while he discharges blood from both nostrils, he suffers with stiffness in the neck, and he is speechless." (Critchley, 1970, p. 55).

Approximately 800 years later in the *Gloss,* an account of the passage, more detail was given about the patient's neurogenic communication disorder and that his speechlessness was caused by a projectile-induced open head injury. According to O'Neill (1980), the ancient Egyptians did not believe the patient's fundamental nature was altered by the injury nor were his symptoms caused by an irrational element. They recognized the relationship between the brain and the ability to speak, and that brain damage could cause speechlessness. However, the ancient Egyptians believed the heart was the seat of the soul and center for life-memories (Bear, Connors, and Paradiso, 1998).

The Chinese developed acupuncture in 2500 B.C. (Scientific American, 1999). Acupuncture is the procedure of using long thin needles to achieve various body states including anesthesia.

The Ancient Greeks and Romans

The ancient Greek philosophers furthered the study of neurogenic communication disorders by addressing the *brain-mind leap.* Hippocrates, the father of medicine, advanced the idea that the brain is where thought is found in the human body and consequently connected brain damage to cognitive impairments. Hippocrates also broke from the irrational beliefs of the time, particularly that illness was punishment from the gods for bad deeds and that offenders would be cured by pleasing them. Hippocrates was a believer in *body humors,* that a healthy body had a balance of the four humors: blood, black bile, yellow bile, and phlegm, and having these humors out-of-balance caused illness. By logical extension, Hippocrates believed that an imbalance of body humors could cause neurogenic communication disorders. Hippocrates introduced the terms *aphonos* and *anaudos* for neurogenic communication disorders (Benton, 1981). Treatments based on the *body humors theory* included inducing vomiting and bloodletting. The humor theory of illness was practiced in one form or another into the 1700s.

Plato, Socrates, and Aristotle philosophized about thought, thinking, and emotions. Plato and Socrates considered thought to be a "conversation" with the soul. Plato believed that the bloodstream conducted sound to the ear and that hearing was the exact reverse of speech production. Socrates dictum, "know thyself," addressed the thought-language controversy, and looked to language as a means of self-exploration. While Aristotle believed that the heart, not the brain, was the center for many sensations and motor functions, he set the groundwork for the scientific exploration of neurogenic communication disorders. He introduced words to describe anatomic and physiologic concepts such as *category, form,* and *principle* (Bois, 1966). Aristotle philosophized about neurogenic communication disorders and addressed several speech impediments (O'Neill, 1980). He wrote about the speech of drunken persons, articulation irregularities resulting from excessive cold, stroke, and the speech of depressed persons. Aristotle coined the terms *ischnophonos* (hesitancy in speech), *traylos* (lisping), and *psellos* (stammering) although the terms do not correspond to modern definitions (O'Neill, 1980).

> According to Benton and Joynt (1960), Valerius Maximus (Circa A.D. 30) first described a case of alexia that was of traumatic origins.

Galen, a surgeon to the gladiators, wrote extensively about anatomy and believed in the body humors theory of illness. Galen thought that nature was an expression of a divine spirit and understood the value of studying diseases and disorders as a way of learning about normal functions (Scientific American, 1999). He believed that the *cerebrum* was the recipient of sensation and the *cerebellum* the command center for muscular movement (Bear, Connors, and Paradiso, 1998). While Galen was not a Christian, he believed that communication was "God-given," and that its disorders were divine impositions.

The Middle Ages and Renaissance

The *Dark Ages* began at the end of the Roman Empire and lasted nearly 600 years. According to Lum (2002), nothing of significance happened intellectually or scientifically in Western civilization during the Dark Ages. However, in other parts of the world, intellectual and scientific thought flourished. In the Western World, the logical reasoning about neurogenic communication disorders during the previous classical period was discarded and replaced by religious dogma. During this time, communication disorders were thought to be punishment from God and the only treatment was through prayer. It was believed that with prayer, God would cure the communication disorder.

During the Dark and *Middle Ages*, superstitions about diseases resulted in brutal treatment for people afflicted with disabilities. In some cities, the disabled dared not go into public places for fear of being stoned (Van Riper and Erickson, 1996). One explanation for the origin of the term "handicapped" comes from the practice of disabled persons begging for food and money with caps extended. Their lives literally depended on the kindness of strangers. Disabled persons were often made scapegoats for the plagues and mass diseases ravaging parts of Europe. Disabled persons were thought to be possessed by evil and Priests and Shaman were used to cast it out.

The *Renaissance* followed the Middle Ages and was a period of rebirth of intellectual curiosity and medical advances. There were major advances in astronomy, physics, and mathematics. In the neurosciences, the body humors theory of body functioning and illness prevailed. However, Rene Descartes proposed that brain mechanisms have limited control for human thought and behavior, and only for animalistic functions: "Descartes believed that the mind is a spiritual entity that receives sensations and commands movements by communicating with the machinery of the brain via the pineal gland" (Bear, Connors, and Paradiso, 1998, p. 6). His belief that the mind is a divine entity reignited the brain-mind dichotomy of mental functions.

During the Renaissance, discussions about neurogenic communication disorders became more detailed and complete. A physician, Antonio Guainerio, described two aphasic patients and detailed their symptoms (Benton and Joynt, 1960). He speculated about the neurological basis to the disorder including an organ of memory and excessive accumulation of phlegm in the fourth ventricle. During this time, some physicians also recognized that brain disease could cause non-paralytic types of communication disorders including loss of memory for words (Benton, 1981).

In 1865, Pierre Paul Broca's famous statement, "We speak with the left hemisphere," harkened an important brain localization period of the study of neurogenic communication disorders. However, before Broca, several investigators postulated functional localized regions in the human brain. The most notable was Franz Joseph Gall. Gall is most remembered for the ill-fated *Phrenology Theory* and that a person's mental and personality traits could be discovered by palpations of the bones of the skull. However, Gall's contribution to neuroscience went beyond the ill-conceived pseudoscience of phrenology. According to Benson and Ardilla (1996), Gall ranks among the foremost neuroanatomists of his day and he categorized human brain function into a vital force, inclinations of the soul, and intellectual qualities of the mind. Notably, he postulated that verbal and grammatical memory was localized to convolutions of the brain.

Pierre Paul Broca and Karl Wernicke

Based on postmortem examinations of aphasic patients who had been under his care, Pierre Paul Broca localized expressive speech and language to the third frontal convolution of the left hemisphere. Broca labeled the loss of the ability to combine articulatory movements into words as *aphemia* (aphemie). He also identified *amnesie verbale* as a disorder in which the patient pronounces words correctly, but has lost the ability to associate ideas with words (Benson and Ardilla, 1996). Especially among physicians, *Broca's area* has become synonymous with the expressive speech and language center of the brain, and *Broca's aphasia* is a general clinical term for expressive motor speech and language disorders.

> Pierre Paul Broca was born in 1824 and died in 1880. He graduated from medical school when he was just 20 years-old.

At about the same time Broca was localizing the expressive speech and language centers of the brain, a German physician, Karl Wernicke, identified the receptive language area to the left hemisphere. Wernicke's area, now synonymous with the site of the brain considered responsible for auditory comprehension, is in the posterior, superior gyrus of the temporal lobe. However, some present-day authorities also extend it into the adjacent parietal lobe, especially when addressing reading comprehension. For example, Zemlin (1998) shows Wernicke's area extending into the parietal lobe. Especially among physicians, *Wernicke's aphasia*, sometimes called *sensory aphasia*, is a general term for receptive speech and language impairments.

Karl Wernicke was born in Poland in 1848 and died in 1905. He received his medical training in Germany.

Wernicke is noted for providing the first detailed classification system for neurogenic communication disorders based on anatomical and pathological localizations. According to Sies (1974), Wernicke postulated three types of aphasia besides *sensory aphasia,* localized in the first temporal convolution, which may result in jargon and the inability to understand speech. He labeled Broca's "amnesie verbale" as *motor aphasia* and reported that these patients could understand speech but only produce a few words. *Total aphasia* was characterized as a severe expressive and receptive speech and language impairment. Wernicke also postulated a new type of aphasia resulting from damage to the pathways between the anterior motor and posterior sensory regions of the brain. This language disorder is presently called *conduction aphasia* (Benson and Ardilla, 1996). According to Love and Webb (2001, p. 6), "Wernicke organized the symptoms of language disturbance in such a way that they could be used diagnostically to predict the lesion site in either connective pathways or centers in the language system."

The Holistic Theorists

A hotly contested debate about the study of normal speech and language functioning and neurogenic communication disorders erupted during the latter part of the 1800s and continues today. On one side of the issue are the *localizationists* who believe that speech and language functions and disorders can be understood by examining sites, centers, or networks of the brain and the effects of damage to them.

Most reports were observations of language function made during the life of the patient and ascribed to a neuroanatomical locus of pathology demonstrated at postmortem. The psychological findings were expressed in the jargon of the day, and with few exceptions the anatomical descriptions involved the cortical surface only. Selected cortical areas were proposed as "centers," essential for a specific language function (although some investigators were aware of and even described networks). Proposed centers included such entities as a gleidokinetic center, a writing center, an auditory-verbal image center, a center for symbols, a center for object images, and numerous others. (Benson and Ardilla, 1996, p. 16)

Criticism of the localization movement regarding speech and language functions centered on isolation of the specific sites and neuronal tracts of the brain and whether pure and absolute neurogenic communication disorders exit.

Pierre Marie, a French neurologist, voiced early opposition to Broca's localization discovery. Marie argued against an expressive speech and language center in the left hemisphere in a series of scientific papers based on reexamination of the brains of Broca's first two patients (Benson and Ardilla, 1996). As reported in Chapter 1, neurologist Sir Henry Head, a graduate of Cambridge University, was an outspoken critic of the brain localization movement. In his 1926 book, *Aphasia and Kindred Disorders of Speech,* he sarcastically labeled localizationists as *diagram makers*. Head criticized Wernicke for his lack of scientific objectivity, a tendency to "lop and twist" clinical manifestations from hypothetical brain lesions, and his lack of scientific insight (Sies, 1974).

Henry Head also postulated four broad categories of aphasia based on linguistic deficits. His categorization system avoided the pure expressive-receptive dichotomy popular at the time. According to Eisenson (1984), Head's *verbal aphasia* mainly affects words as parts of a phrase and includes defective articulatory and auditory functions. *Syntactical aphasia* is essentially a disorder of balance and rhythm of speech and involves defective grammar. *Nominal aphasia* is loss of the ability to comprehend the meaning of words and other symbols, and *semantic aphasia* is primarily the loss of verbal intellect.

Neurologist John Hughlings Jackson developed the concept of *inner speech* (internal monologues) and the *proposition* as the fundamental unit of speech. What is most important, Jackson formally addressed the role of the patient's *psyche* in communication and its disorders.

> To speak is not simply to utter words, it is to propositionise. A proposition is such a relation of words that it makes one new meaning; not by a mere addition of what we call the separate meanings of the several words; the terms of the proposition are modified by each other. Single words are meaningless, and so is any unrelated succession of words. The unit of speech is the proposition. A single word is, or is in effect, a proposition, if other words in relation are implied (Jackson, 1878, p. 311).

According to Sies (1974), Jackson believed that inner speech occurs with the same structure as other propositional utterances and that it was artificial to consider externalized language as fundamentally different from internal monologues.

> John Hughlings Jackson fused thought, language, and the individual's intent in communicating to the study of neurogenic communication disorders.

Similar to other holistic theorists, neurologist Theodore Weisenburg and psychologist Katharine E. McBride developed a classification system for aphasia that did not include the absolute *expressive-receptive dichotomy* and the existence of pure types of aphasia. Weisenberg and McBride (1935) systematically studied hospitalized aphasic patients with several neuropsychological tests and advanced the idea of *predominantly* expressive and receptive aphasia:

> *Predominantly expressive aphasia*: The greatest amount of disturbance is with verbal or written expression.

Predominantly receptive aphasia: The greatest amount of disturbance is with the comprehension of spoken and/ or written symbols.

Amnesic aphasia: Primary deficit is the evocation of words for expression.

Expressive-receptive aphasia: Extreme disturbance in both verbal and graphic expression and reception.

Some authorities on neurogenic communication disorders consider Weisenberg and McBride's research as the first true scientific examination of aphasia and related disorders. Unfortunately, their conclusions about the performance of aphasic subjects were questionable because of flawed research design; their subjects were not neurologically stable at the time of testing. Despite the weakness of the research design, Weisenberg and McBride's observed that receptive functions are more likely to resolve spontaneously (Eisenson, 1984). Schuell, Jenkins, and Jimenez-Pabon (1964, p. 44) summarize their study as timeless: "Good clinical observations are never dated and in this respect this is a timeless study." Their classification system served as a model for Eisenson's *Examining for Aphasia*, a popular clinical test during the latter part of the 1900s.

Joseph Wepman (1962) believes aphasia is a *psycholinguistic regression* and that it affects the patient's entire personality. Accordingly, the speechlessness of an infant corresponds to global aphasia and the stage of language acquisition where there is learning of vocabulary correlates with semantic aphasia. Aphasias affecting syntactic processing correlate with the grammatical acquisition stages in children. Wepman and Jones (1961) propose that stages of recovery from aphasia should parallel the stages of language acquisition.

> According to Wepman (1962, p. 207), the aphasic patient must reorganize his or her self-concept: "The self-concept evolved must be in terms of the patient as he is, facing the reality of his condition and leaving the 'ghost of the past' that so often haunts him."

The *language-thought controversy* is apparent in Wepman's view of aphasia. Wepman (1976, p. 131) notes: "When cortical impairment produces an observable linguistic deficiency, the disturbance may lie in the language structure and form of expression or it may lie in the limitation of the underlying thought processes thereby affecting linguistic expression." Kurt Goldstein also addressed the language-thought controversy. Goldstein postulated an *abstract-concrete imbalance* in aphasic patients' performance of reasoning tasks and the loss of an *abstract attitude*. This loss of abstract attitude was present in language and nonverbal performance tasks such as classifying objects and sorting colors (Goldstein, 1959, 1952, 1948, 1924).

The Russian psychologist, Aleksandr R. Luria, views neurogenic communication disorders based on *Pavlovian psychology* and took exception with Wepman's psycholinguistic regression theory (1974, 1970, 1966, 1964, 1958). He suggests that the effects of learning and experience are very strong in adults and that brain damage does not return the individual to stages of development he or she has previously passed. The aphasic patient's previous experiences cannot leave him or her unchanged, even after extensive brain damage. According to Luria, the human experience is a process of transformation which leaves the adult unique and psychologically different from the child.

> According to Davis (2007), Luria divided the central nervous system into three divisions: general and sensory awareness, perception and interpretation of sensory information, and volitional responses.

Luria proposed several unique ways of understanding aphasia and related disorders. Fundamental to his system was the notion of *analysis*, the breakup of a signal into its basic elements, and *synthesis*, combining its components. Disorders affecting analysis of the speech signal involves the patient's ability to breakdown speech and language into meaningful elements. Synthesis, on the other hand, is the ability to synthesize the communicative intent into speech and language. Another unique contribution to the classification of neurogenic communication disorders by Luria involves cognitive-linguistic disturbance and a breakdown in the patient's internal speech. He labeled the various disorders *sensory, acoustic-amnestic, afferent* (kinesthetic) *motor, efferent* (kinetic) *motor, semantic,* and *dynamic aphasias.*

Roman Jakobson (1964) and Jakobson and Halle (1956) took a linguistic approach to aphasia classification and reconciled Luria's system by combining efferent, afferent and dynamic aphasia into *contiguity* disorders and a deterioration of context. *Similarity* disorders involved damage to the speech and language code and included sensory, amnestic, and semantic disorders. Although Luria was a vocal opponent of the localization movement, he tied several of his categories to specific brain lesions. Schuell, Jenkins, and Jimenez-Pabon (1964, p. 53) summarize Luria's neuroanatomic correlates of aphasia:

> To summarize Luria's theory of aphasia: a lesion in Wernicke's area results in an impairment of phonemic discrimination, which affects articulation, vocabulary, and writing. A lesion in the parietal or parieto-occipital area results in a disturbance of simultaneous synthesis, reflected in inability to synthesize parts into wholes, difficulty in arithmetic and in comprehending and communicating relationships expressed through the logico-grammatical forms of language. A lesion in the fronto-temporal area causes a disturbance in sequential synthesis, primarily affecting communication of events, and characterized by impairment of syntactical usage, of internal speech, and fluency.

Hildred Schuell classified aphasia based on groupings and severity of symptoms which served as the basis for her popular test: *The Minnesota Test for the Differential Diagnosis of Aphasia* (Schuell, 1955). Although Schuell advanced the understanding of aphasia and related disorders, especially for rehabilitation purposes, she further complicated the aphasia classification controversy by introducing perceptual, sensorimotor, visual, and dysarthric components to her five "groups" of patients. Schuell postulated that language is the central disorder of aphasia and that the most severe type of aphasia is irreversible. Jenkins, Jimenez-Pabon, Shaw, and Sefer (1975) added *prosodic disturbance* and *intermittent auditory-acoustic agnosia* to Schuell's original five categories.

> In 1970, Hildred Schuell received "The Honors of the Association" for distinguished contribution to the field of speech, language, and hearing by the American Speech-Language-Hearing Association.

Constantin von Monakow, Macdonald Critchley, and Russell Brain addressed the importance of the psychological factors in a *holistic* view of neurogenic communication disorders. Von Monakow believed that there is no aphasia, only aphasic patients, and that large and variable surrounding areas of brain damage accompany all cerebral pathology (Benson, 1979). Critchley (1970) explored the use of inner symbols in aphasia and postulated the existence of a *grammar to inner speech*. Brain (1965) concluded that aphasia is more than a neurological event; it must be considered on a psychological level.

John Sarno (1981) addresses etiology and a holistic view of neurogenic communication disorders and suggests a logical set of ground rules for a *science of emotions*. Categorical separation of groups for study should include " . . . patients with unilateral stroke (with the lesion in the distribution of one vessel only), space-occupying tumors, invasive tumors, missile wounds, head trauma with focal lesions (lacerations, loss of substance, intracerebral hemorrhage, peridural hemorrhage), head trauma without focal lesions and with coma" (J. Sarno, 1981, pg. 481).

Jon Eisenson has been a leader in holistic view of neurogenic communication disorders especially as it relates to the patient's personality. "We would consider it surprising if an individual who has incurred a cerebral insult and associated aphasic disturbances did not undergo consequent changes in personality" (Eisenson, 1984, p. 87). Eisenson notes that an impairment of language affects the personality especially as it relates to *ego* involvement: "Their inclination, their needs, their interpretations, rather than those of their cultural environment, become the dominant ones (Eisenson, 1984, p. 91). He also notes that aphasic patients have disruptions in the capacity for planning acknowledging Goldstein's observations that aphasic patients have *loss of abstract attitude*. According to Eisenson, those who make expected good recoveries adjust to the brain damage, and those who do not reach their potential are hindered by their premorbid inclinations and ego involvement.

The New Localizationists

In the mid 1900s, Norman Geschwind challenged the holistic view of neurogenic communication disorders and returned to a *neuroanatomical-psychological correlation theory* (Benson and Ardilla, 1996). In a series of papers, he introduced a *cortical disconnection* theory to explain the symptoms of neurogenic communication disorders. He concentrated on *dyslexia* and other developmental neurological disorders. According to Geschwind, the disconnection syndromes resulted from lesions isolating cortical and subcortical functional centers. He also addressed the variety of naming errors in aphasia. According to Geschwind (1971, 1967), *nonfluent aphasia*, associated with damage to Broca's area, is uttered slowly, results in little productive speech, and is often telegraphic. He also identified several types of *fluent aphasia* and their neuroanatomical sites of lesions. Fluent aphasia has normal grammatical skeleton and prosody and results from the habitual use of circumlocutions, paraphasias, and nonspecific words. "His combination of pertinent clinical observations, superb scholarship, and vigorous presentation of a rational scientific-philosophic approach won the day" (Benson and Ardilla, 1996, p. 21).

The *Boston Classification System* links neuroanatomical sites of lesions and aphasia, and serves as the basis for the *Boston Diagnostic Aphasia Examination* (Goodglass, Kaplan, and Barresi (2001). According to Davis (2007), the third edition of the Boston Diagnostic Aphasia Examination has been extensively revised and classifies aphasia into syndromes according to symptom patterns. Goodglass and Kaplan (1983) also identified two prominent types of aphasia naming errors: *literal* and *verbal paraphasia*. A literal paraphasia is the substituting of a similar sounding word for the desired one, e.g., ton for gun, fat for cat, red for bed. A verbal paraphasia has a semantic relationship to the desired word, e.g., red for blue, top for bottom, dog for cat.

Davis (2007), Murray and Chapey (2001), Eisenson (1984), and Damasio (1981) summarize the syndromes of aphasia identified in the Boston Classification System and the Boston Diagnostic Aphasia Examination. Aphasic patients' language profiles are classified into one of the one of the categories below:

> *Alexia With Agraphia* results in the patient having problems reading and writing, and as a pure syndrome, it is rare.

> *Alexia Without Agraphia,* also called *pure alexia,* results in the patient being unable to read while writing is functional.

> *Anomic Aphasia* is rare and characterized by impairment of word finding in any modality. Repetition and comprehension are intact and the patient is fluent and grammatically correct.

> *Broca's Aphasia* is also called motor or expressive aphasia with nonfluent output, agrammatism, only mild comprehension deficits, and usually associated with right-sided motor deficits.

Conduction Aphasia is limited to the patient's impairment in repeating words and sentences occasionally occurring with minor deficits in aural comprehension.

Global Aphasia, also called total or complete aphasia, affects all modalities of language and limits the patient to a few purposeful words, some serial speech, and emotional utterances.

Pure Word Deafness is the loss of auditory comprehension, complete impairment of repetition, and normally fluent speech mostly without paraphasias.

Transcortical Sensory Aphasia results in fluent, paraphasic speech, intact repetition, and severely compromised auditory comprehension.

Transcortical Motor Aphasia results in nonfluent speech with paraphasia, intact repetition, perseveration, and loss of connective words.

Wernicke's Aphasia is also called sensory or receptive aphasia and combines output and input disturbances, fluent speech that is well articulated with frequent paraphasias, but preserved syntax. Some Wernicke's Aphasia patients produce meaningless jargon output.

Neurologist D. Frank Benson, a leader in the modern localization movement, addresses aphasia, *amnesia, agnosia,* and other neurological disorders by correlating symptoms with brain scans and other neuroanatomical studies. He observes that there is far better agreement on the clinical signs of the syndromes than on their labels (Benson, 1979). Benson (1979) classifies aphasia relative to major brain landmarks and structures. In the current classification system (Benson and Ardila, 1996), cortical involvement syndromes are classified as *pre-Rolandic* or *post-Rolandic* relative to the fissure of Rolando, and Perisylvian or Extrasylvian relative to the fissure of Sylvius.

> Methods of scanning the brain, called neuroimaging, include *computed tomography* (CT), *magnetic resonance imaging* (MRI), *single photon tomography* (SPECT), *positron emission tomography* (PET), and *functional magnetic resonance imaging* (fMRI).

According to Benson and Ardila (1996), pre-Rolandic, Perisylvian area aphasias include *Broca aphasia-type I* and *Broca aphasia-type II*. Broca aphasia-type I is also called *aphemia*, little Broca aphasia, or Broca's area aphasia, and the damage is limited to the cortex and immediate subcortical structures. These patients have only mild articulatory and prosody defects plus reduced wordfinding abilities, and they maintain good language comprehension except for complex utterances. Broca aphasia-type II is based on more extensive brain damage to the opercula, the precentral gyrus, the anterior insula, the periventricular white matter, and/or the white matter deep to the dominant posterior inferior cortex. Broca aphasia-type II is characterized by dysarthria, deficits in the motor activating system, restricted grammar, and lexical deficits.

Pre-Rolandic, Extrasylvian area aphasias include *Extrasylvian motor aphasia-type I* and *Extrasylvian motor aphasia-type II*. Extrasylvian (transcortical) motor aphasia-type I is characterized by disordered nonfluent verbal output and good comprehension. Repetition of spoken language is good and this type of aphasia is also known as dynamic aphasia, loss of verbal initiative, and transcortical motor aphasia. It results from damage to the left dorsolateral prefrontal area. Extrasylavian (transcortical) motor aphasia-type II is also known as transcortical motor aphasia, syndrome of the anterior cerebral artery, mild transcortical motor aphasia, and supplementary motor area aphasia. Clinical aspects of Extrasylavian (transcortical) motor aphasia-type II include good repetition and comprehension of spoken language, sparse effortful conversational language, occasional literal paraphasia, and impaired reading and writing.

Post-Rolandic language area aphasias include conduction aphasia resulting from damage to the parietal-insular area, Wernicke aphasia-type I resulting from damage to the posterior insular-temporal isthmus, and Wernicke aphasia-type II, damage to the superior and middle temporal gyri. Conduction aphasia, primarily a repetition abnormality, is also known as central aphasia, efferent conduction aphasia, and repetition conduction aphasia. It results from disconnection of the language comprehension from the production areas and tracts. Wernicke aphasia-type I is also known as acoustic-agnosia aphasia, word-deafness, and verbal auditory agnosia. Wernicke aphasia-type II features a greater degree of word-blindness than word-deafness. Besides alexia, these patients also have impairments with auditory comprehension and repetition of spoken language.

Post-Rolandic language area aphasias include Extrasylvian (transcortical) sensory aphasia-type I, resulting from damage to the junction of the temporal, parietal, and occipital lobes. Extrasylvian sensory aphasia-type II is caused by damage to the parieto-occipital lobes and the angular gyrus. Extrasylvian sensory aphasia-type I is also known as amnesic aphasia and is characterized by fluent spontaneous language, preserved repetition, and poor comprehension. Echolalia, neologistic substitutions, and semantic paraphasia are also present. Extrasylvian (transcortical) sensory aphasia-type II is also called semantic and anomic aphasia, and patients have difficulty integrating the elements of a sentence into a whole and grasping the meaning of relationships. Benson and Ardila (1996) also describe mixed varieties of aphasia.

Previously described aphasias include *borderzone, subcortical,* and *nonlocalizing syndromes* (Benson, 1979). Borderzone aphasia syndromes result from infarcts in the areas served by the middle cerebral artery and those of the anterior or posterior cerebral arteries. Borderzone aphasia includes mixed, and transcortical motor and sensory aphasia. Subcortical aphasia, a controversial category, may result from damage to the thalamus. Global aphasia is considered a nonlocalizing aphasic syndrome.

Aphasia Without Adjectives

In 1982, Frederic L. Darley, published his landmark text, *Aphasia*, revolutionizing the study of neurogenic communication disorders. It was preceded by the equally influential book *Motor Speech Disorders* (Darley, Aronson, and Brown, 1975). These two textbooks simplified the complex and often confusing categorization system of neurogenic communication disorders by clearly distinguishing the motor speech disorders of apraxia of speech and the dysarthrias from the language disorder of aphasia.

Darley's approach to classifying aphasia involves three important distinctions leading to the concept of *aphasia without adjectives*. The first distinction is that *aphasia is not a speech disorder.* "Aphasia is a language problem, not a speech problem. It is not the result of difficulties in either the programming or the execution of certain muscular movements. It does not relate to any dysfunction in the basic motor speech processes, the mechanics of exteriorizing ideas through speech. Rather, it has to do with how efficiently one processes the symbolic code that constitutes language" (Darley, 1982, p. 8). Aphasia is a distinct disorder separate from motor speech disorders. In motor speech disorders, the patient has good command of language.

> In 1967, Canter classified motor speech disorders as either central or peripheral. In the central category, he listed *spastic, dyskinetic,* and *ataxic neuromotor* speech disorders. In the peripheral category, he listed *myopathic, myoneural* and *lower motor neuron neuromotor* disorders.

Research conducted at the Mayo Clinic in Rochester, Minnesota served as the basis for delineating the different types of motor speech disorders. In the study, 212 subjects were used with seven types of neurogenic communication disorders: pseudobulbar palsy, bulbar palsy, amyotrophic lateral sclerosis, cerebellar lesions, parkinsonism, dystonia, and chorea. Based on this research, Darley, Aronson, and Brown (1975) differentiated between *apraxia of speech*, a speech programming and execution disorder, and six dysarthrias: *flaccid, spastic, ataxic, hypokinetic, hyperkinetic,* and *mixed*.

The second distinction is that *aphasia is language-specific* and addresses the language-thought controversy. According to Darley (1982, p. 22), "The aphasic patient's difficulty is in the processing of the language code, however received or expressed, whether by listening, reading, speaking, writing, or gesturing, and this dysfunction is disproportionate to dysfunction in other cognitive areas." However, Darley recognizes that aphasic patients suffer from reduced intelligence due to the role language plays in thought and a general reduction in the ability to abstract.

Darley's third distinction is that *aphasia is not modality-bound*. "The concept most in accord with the facts is that aphasia is a multimodality symbolic disorder resulting from malfunction of a central integrative mechanism not bound to any particular transmission channel–of ingress or egress–but making use of and relating to all of them" (Darley, 1982, pp. 28-29). With this distinction, he acknowledges an integral and central unifying language processing function.

Darley (1982) proposed designating patients as aphasic without adjectives and thus solving the age-old classification problem. Aphasia without adjectives recognizes that previous classification systems of aphasia often included associated disorders and that patients distribute themselves on a continuum of severity. What is most important, Darley acknowledges that labeling aphasic disorders is often self-defeating because most patients significantly evolve overtime in their symptoms rendering firm and stable classification impossible.

Neurogenic Communication Disorders in the 21st Century

Centuries have transpired since the ancient Egyptian's pondered the relationship between speech and the brain, the effects of brain damage on the ability to speak, and how neurogenic communication disorders affect the patient's heart, mind, and soul. While there have been many advances in the neurosciences and neurogenic communication disorders, some issues that surfaced about 4000 years ago continue to challenge current scientists and clinicians. Modern scientists and clinicians wrestle with many of the same issues faced by their ancient Egyptian, Greek, and Roman counterparts. Important theoretical and clinical issues that remain include the brain-mind leap, localization of communication functions, thought and language, labeling and categorizing systems for aphasia and related disorders, efficacy of treatment, and the patient's adjustment to the neurogenic communication disorders.

Today, while it is recognized that thought occurs in the brain, not the heart as the as the ancient physicians believed, projecting the workings of the brain to what occurs in a person's mind still challenges scientists and clinicians. Integral to the brain-mind leap is the role of language in cognition: Does language simply express thought? A problem that plagued scientists and clinicians throughout the ages, and continues today, is a lack of definition uniformity and many disparate categorization systems for neurogenic communication disorders. Throughout history and today, philosophers, scientists, and clinicians have little agreement about clinical terms and their meanings for neurogenic communication disorders. Even today, like the ancient Egyptian physicians, a few authorities question the efficacy of treatment for neurogenic communication disorders in general, and for particularly types of impairments. A current issue, first addressed 4000 years ago, continues today: How do patients adjust to neurogenic communication disorders and how do they affect their quality of life?

The study and treatment of neurogenic communication disorders have rarely been free from controversy. In fact, Benson (1993) reports that the discipline of aphasiology was born from the long simmering debate over localized versus holistic explanations of the functions in the brain. Heilman and Valenstein (1993) note that there are many valid approaches to the study of the brain and no morally and intellectually sound ones should be neglected. The study and treatment of neurogenic communication disorders have a long history of intellectual curiosity and heated debate. The 21st Century will no doubt be a remarkable time of scientific, philosophical, and clinical advances in the study and treatment of neurogenic communication disorders.

Chapter Summary

The study and treatment of neurogenic communication disorders have a long and exciting history. The ancient Egyptians, Greeks, and Romans studied the brain, nervous system, and neurogenic communication disorders setting the foundation for many topics currently being examined. Scientists and clinicians throughout history have pondered important issues related to neurogenic communication disorders such as the brain-mind dichotomy, localized and holistic theories about language functions and communication disorders, and classification systems. The effects of language disorders on intelligence and cognition, and the influence of neurogenic communication disorders on the patient's personality, continue to be studied, discussed, and debated. The study and treatment of neurogenic communication disorders will continue to be a rich source of information about human brain and nervous system functioning into the 21st Century.

Study and Discussion Questions

1. Why study the history of neurogenic communication disorders?
2. What did the ancient Egyptians believe about the brain, nervous system, and brain damage?
3. What did the ancient Greeks and Romans believe about thought, thinking, and emotions?
4. What happened during the Middle Ages and the Renaissance regarding the study and treatment of neurogenic communication disorders?
5. What were Pierre Paul Broca's and Karl Wernicke's contributions to the study of aphasia and related disorders?

6. Compare and contrast the "diagram makers" and "holistic theorists."

7. Discuss inner speech (internal monologues) and propositional utterances.

8. Is aphasia a psycholinguistic regression? Defend your position.

9. Describe the contributions of the new localizationists to the study and treatment of neurogenic communication disorders.

10. What is meant by "aphasia without adjectives?"

References

Bear, M. F., Connors, B.W., and Paradiso, M.A. (1998). *Neuroscience: Exploring the brain.* Baltimore: Williams & Wilkins.

Benson, F. D. (1979). *Aphasia, alexia, and agraphia.* New York: Churchill Livingstone.

Benson, F. D. (1993). Aphasia. In *Clinical neuropsychology.* K. Heilman and E. Valenstein (Eds). New York: Oxford University Press.

Benson, F. D. and Ardila, A. (1996). *Aphasia: A clinical perspective.* New York: Oxford University Press.

Benton, A. (1981). Aphasia: Historical perspectives. In M. Sarno (Ed), *Acquired aphasia.* New York: Academic Press.

Benton, A. and Joynt, R. (1960). Early descriptions of aphasia. *Archives of Neurology*, 3: 205-221.

Bois, J. S. (1966). *The art of awareness: A textbook on general semantics.* Dubuque, IA: William C. Brown.

Brain, R. (1965). *Speech disorders: Aphasia, apraxia and agnosia* (2nd ed.). Washington, DC: Butterworth.

Canter, G. (1967). Neuromotor pathologies of speech. *American Journal of Physical Medicine*, 46: 569.

Critchley, M. (1970). *Aphasiology and other aspects of language.* London, UK: Edward Arnold.

Damasio, A. (1981). The nature of aphasia: Signs and syndromes. In *Acquired aphasia.* M. Sarno (Ed). New York: Academic Press.

Darley, F.L. (1982). *Aphasia.* Philadelphia: W.B. Saunders.

Darley, F., Aronson, A., and Brown, J. (1975). *Motor speech disorders.* Philadelphia: W. B. Saunders.

Davis, G.A. (2007). *Aphasiology: Disorders and clinical practice* (2nd ed.) Boston: Pearson, Allyn and Bacon.

Eisenson, J. (1984). *Adult aphasia* (2nd ed.). Englewood Cliffs, N.J.: Prentice-Hall.

Geschwind, N. (1967). The varieties of naming errors. *Cortex*, 3 (1): 97-112.

Geschwind, N. (1971). Aphasia. *New England Journal of Medicine*, 284: 654-656.

Goldstein, K. (1924). Das wesen der amnestischen aphasia. *Schweizer Archiv fuer Neurologia and Psychiatrie*, 15: 163-175.

Goldstein, K. (1948). *Language and language disturbances.* New York: Grune and Stratton.

Goldstein, K. (1952). The effects of brain damage on the personality. *Psychiatry*, 15: 245-260.

Goldstein, K. (1959). Functional disturbances in the brain. In *American handbook of psychiatry*, S. Arieti (Ed). New York: Basic Books.

Goodglass, H. and Kaplan, E. (1983). *The assessment of aphasia and other neurological disorders.* Baltimore, MD: Williams and Wilkins.

Goodglass, H. Kaplan, E., and Barresi, B. (2001). *The assessment of aphasia and related disorders* (3rd ed.). Philadelphia: Lippincott, Williams, & Wilkins.

Head, H. (1926). *Aphasia and kindred disorders of speech.* New York: Cambridge University Press and Macmillian. (Reprinted in 1963 by Hafner Publishing Co., New York).

Heilman, K. and Valenstein, E. (1993). Introduction. In *Clinical neuropsychology.* K. Heilman and E. Valenstein (Eds). New York: Oxford University Press.

Jakobson, R. (1964). Toward a linguistic typology of aphasic impairments. In *Disorders of language.* A. DeReuck and M. O'Connor (Eds). London: J. & A. Churchill.

Jakobson, R. and Halle, M. (1956) *Fundamentals of language.* The Hague: Mouton.

Jackson, J. (1878). On affections of speech from diseases of the brain. *Brain.* 1: 301-330.

Jenkins, J., Jimenez-Pabon, I., Shaw, R., and Sefer, J. (1975). *Schuell's aphasia in adults* (2nd ed.). New York: Harper and Row.

Luria, A. (1958). Brain disorders and language analysis. *Language and speech,* 1: 14-34.

Luria, A. (1964). Factors and Forms of Aphasia. In *Disorders of language.* A. DeReuck and M. O'Connor (Eds). London: J. & A. Churchill.

Luria, A. (1966). *Higher cortical function in man.* New York: Basic Books.

Luria, A. (1970). *Traumatic aphasia: Its syndromes, psychology and treatment.* The Hague: Mouton.

Luria, A. (1974). Language and brain. *Brain and Language*, 1: 1-14.

Lum, C. (2002). *Scientific thinking in speech and language therapy.* Mahwah, New Jersey: Lawrence Erlbaum Associates.

Love, R. J. and Webb, W.G. (2001). Neurology for the speech-language pathologist (4th ed.). Boston: Butterworth-Heinemann.

Murray, L.L. and Chapey, R. (2001). Assessment of language disorders in adults. In *Language intervention in aphasia and related neurogenic communication disorders* (4th ed.). R. Chapey (Ed). Philadelphia: Lippincott Williams and Wilkins.

O'Neill, Y.V. (1980). *Speech and speech disorders in western thought before 1600.* Westport, Connecticut: Greenwood Press.

Sarno, J. (1981). Emotional aspects of aphasia. In *Acquired aphasia.* M. Sarno (Ed), New York: Academic Press.

Schuell, H. (1955). *Minnesota test for the differential diagnosis of aphasia.* Minneapolis: University of Minnesota Press.

Schuell, H., Jenkins, J., and Jimenez-Pabon, E. (1964). *Aphasia in adults.* New York: Harper and Row.

Scientific American Science Desk Reference (1999). New York: John Wiley & Sons.

Sies, L. (1974). *Aphasia: Theory and therapy.* Baltimore: University Park Press.

Van Riper, C., & Erickson, R. (1996). *Speech correction* (9th ed.). Boston: Allyn & Bacon.

Wepman, J. (1962). The language disorders. In J. F. Garrett and E. S. Levine (Eds). *Psychological practices with the physically disabled.* New York: Colombia University Press.

Wepman, J. (1976). Aphasia: Language without thought or thought without language? *Journal of the American Speech and Hearing Association*, 18: 131-136.

Wepman, J. and Jones, L. (1961). *Studies in aphasia: An approach to testing.* Chicago: University of Chicago.

Chapter Three: Aphasia

"Aphasia is a language problem,
not a speech problem."

Frederic L. Darley

Chapter Preview: This chapter defines aphasia and provides the essential linguistic parameters of the definition of this neurogenic communication disorder. There is a discussion of common diagnostic terms used to label aphasic disorders. The language encoding and decoding disorders of aphasia are defined, described, and discussed. Additional topics addressed in this chapter include agrammatism, acalculia, and aphasia in multilingual persons. The value and efficacy of aphasia therapy are reviewed including the principles for optimal aphasia therapy.

The Devastation of Aphasia

Language is essential to the human experience and gives richness to living. For most people, aphasia, loss of the ability to speak, read, write, gesture, and understand the speech of others, is nearly impossible to fathom because language is second-nature. "When an adult suddenly loses the easy use of language, it is a devastating experience for the individual and for the family. Aphasia, and other adult language disorders, affect that which makes us uniquely human– our ability to communicate with each other by a system of language symbols" (Haynes and Pindzola, 2004, p. 219). It is not surprising that aphasia can be disabling on many levels. To make matters worse, aphasia usually has a rapid onset, leaving the patient with little time to prepare for the major life-changes it will bring. Even if the patient could prepare, most persons only have a vague understanding of this complicated neurogenic communication disorder. Unless a person has a friend or relative with aphasia, much of what he or she knows about it is usually a product of the motion picture industry. While Hollywood does a commendable job addressing many communication disorders, it deals with aphasia simplistically often with broad stereotypes and inaccurate depictions of its clinical symptoms (Tanner, 2003a; Tanner, 2001; Tanner, Culbertson, and Secord, 2001).

Psychologically, aphasia is a *double-edged sword* slicing deeply into a person's *quality of life*. Aphasia impairs the patient's ability to communicate with family, friends, and medical professionals separating him or her from people who can and want to help. Aphasia also affects the patient's lifelong *coping styles, verbal defense mechanisms*, and the disorder itself, is a *grievous* event (Tanner, 2009; Tanner and Cotton, 2005; Tanner, 2003b). Of course, there are some individuals with mild aphasia, which is largely an inconvenience, and those who suffer only temporary loss of language, but unfortunately, these are exceptions. While some scientists and clinicians distinguish between "aphasia" as the total loss of language, and "dysphasia" as a milder form of the disorder, most persons refer to the acquired loss of language, no matter its severity, as simply "aphasia." In this book, "mild," "moderate," and "severe" will be used to express degrees of aphasia and its clinical manifestations.

Defining Aphasia

As reported in Chapter 2, throughout history, vague clinical terminology, disparate classification systems, and controversies about its fundamental nature have plagued the study of aphasia. Wertz (2000, p. 6) observes: "Aphasiology's past has provided a variety of definitions of aphasia; new ones emerge frequently; and the future, probably, will perpetuate the practice." Today, there is an evolving consensus about the important parameters of aphasia and what should be included and excluded in its study. Before addressing the essential parameters of aphasia, it is necessary clearly to define the disorder. It should be noted that on a fundamental level, aphasia is essentially *amnesia* for words and all definitions expand on that notion.

> "Despite the tremendous frustration and alteration in *self-concept* that aphasia produces, most of our clients have not exhibited much change in their basic personality traits" (Haynes and Pindzola, 2004, p. 242).

Chapey and Hallowell (2001, p. 3) briefly define aphasia as " . . . an acquired communication disorder caused by brain damage, characterized by an impairment of language modalities: speaking, listening, reading and writing . . . " They go on to note that it is not the result of psychiatric disorders, general intellectual deficits, or sensory impairments. Davis' (2007, p. 15) definition of aphasia omits references to etiology: "Aphasia is a selective impairment of the cognitive system specialized for comprehending and formulating language, leaving other cognitive capacities relatively intact." Darley's (1982, p. 42) definition is the most comprehensive:

> *Aphasia:* Impairment, as a result of brain damage, of the capacity for interpretation and formulation of language symbols; multimodality loss or reduction in efficiency of the ability to decode and encode conventional meaningful linguistic elements (morphemes and larger syntactic units); disproportionate to impairment of other intellective functions; not attributable to dementia, confusion, sensory loss, or motor dysfunction; and manifest in reduced availability of vocabulary, reduced efficiency in application of syntactic rules, reduced auditory retention span, and impaired efficiency in input and output channel selection.

Given such multifaceted perspectives on aphasia, what are the essential elements of a definition of this neurogenic communication disorder?

To reflect current understanding of aphasia, there are four essential parameters to any definition of this neurogenic communication disorder. First, aphasia is a disorder of language *symbolism* and not a speech pathology. Second, aphasia involves *encoding* (synthesis) and *decoding* (analysis) of language codes. Third, aphasia is *multimodality;* it affects, more or less, all avenues of language expression and reception. Fourth, aphasia disproportionately impairs *verbal thought processes* relative to other cognitive processes. Because aphasia is a language disorder, there are essential linguistic parameters included in any definition of aphasia.

Essential Parameters of Language in the Definition of Aphasia

Language is symbolic and aphasia is a symbolic neurogenic communication disorder. A *symbol* is an entity that represents something else. In language, the symbol can be graphic, verbal, or gestural, and that to which it refers is the *referent*. Symbols, by definition, are abstractions; they are generalizations from specific aspects of reality. Vygotsky (1962), a Russian linguist, observes that a word refers to a class of objects rather than a single one, thus generalizing reality differently than an image or other sensation.

Semantics, the substance of language, lies in the symbol-referent relationship and is the foundation to all meaning in language. The symbol-referent relationship is dynamic because language symbols and their meanings change over time. In fact, the meaning of a language symbol changes every time it is used because of the passage of time and the ever-changing nature of reality. Language symbols are also arbitrary; they are randomly created and used by a language community. There are no physical laws or mental requirements that a series of phonemes or graphemes represent a particular entity. Each language community establishes an arbitrary set of symbols to represent reality.

Linguistic *performance* is the use of language in everyday conversation, the user's actual use of language. Linguistic *competence*, possessed by native users of a language, is the knowledge of the language codes. *Grammar* is a general term for the rules of the form and usage of a language. Contrary to the arbitrary nature of semantics, grammar gives stability, predictability, form, and order to language. According to Campbell (1982, p. 165), "Grammar which is part of [language] competence, acts as a filter screening out errors and incorrect arrangements of words, showing a speaker which sentence forms are admissible, and whether they are connected with certain other sentence forms by rules of transformation."

Expressive language involves encoding thoughts into a linguistic code. This is the process of synthesizing sensory information, perceptions of reality, and thought into linguistic units: *phonology, syntax, semantics,* and *pragmatics.* Phonology is the study of the speech sounds of a language and the way they are combined into syllables and words. Syntax is the linguistic rules for arranging units of meaning into connected utterances. As discussed above, semantics is the meaning of *morphemes,* the smallest units of meaning, words, phrases, and discourse. Expressive language also involves pragmatics and the application of meaning to a particular communicative circumstance or context. Receptive language is the decoding or analyzing of the linguistic units.

There are six primary modes or avenues of communicative expression and reception. Expressively, communicators speak, write, or express themselves with gestures. Receptively, communicators understand what is spoken, read, and decipher expressive gestures. Encoding of thoughts spoken involves speech sound production. Writing is creating meaning with graphemes, and gesturing uses meaningful physical movements to transmit information. Decoding speech is the process of analyzing auditory signals. Reading is the deciphering of graphemes into meaningful linguistic units. Gestural comprehension is the attachment of meaning to gestured physical movements during communication. Mathematics is also a language with expressive and receptive modalities.

In adults, language and abstract thought are fundamentally connected. In young children, language primarily represents thought. Young children are on a concrete level, and words and other utterances reflect what is occurring in their minds. In adults, language not only reflects concrete thought, it is fundamental to abstract thinking. Abstract linguistic constructs such as verbally pondering whether it is ethical to engage in a particular behavior, and processing individual words such as "truthfulness," "inevitable" and "friendship," are cognitive processes that do not derive themselves from tangible objective referents. However, even tangible words and concepts involve abstraction. Sternberg and Ben-Zeev (2001, p. 202) note that even when a person is thinking about the tangible word "chair," he or she also conjures 1) all of the instances of chairs in existence anywhere, 2) instances of chairs that exist only in the imagination, 3) all the characteristics of chairs, 4) all the things that may be done with chairs and, 5) all the other concepts linked to chairs (e.g., things you put on a chair or places where you may find chairs). These abstractions can be viewed as cognitively processing "chairness."

> Cognitive psychology addresses thought, perception, memory, and reason.

Given the above definition requirements for aphasia and the essential elements of language, aphasia is defined as the *multimodality inability or reduced ability to encode, decode, and manipulate symbols for the purposes of verbal thought and/or communication.* This working definition reflects the current understanding of this neurogenic communication disorder and provides a basis for addressing its clinical features. There are five important factors to this definition of aphasia which will be addressed in detail in subsequent sections of this chapter.

First, aphasia is a multimodality neurogenic communication disorder. Although a particular patient may present with predominantly expressive or predominantly receptive symptoms, aphasia, more or less, cuts across all modalities of language. Second, there are degrees of aphasia and the symptoms naturally evolve in type and severity. Third, predominantly expressive aphasia primarily disrupts encoding of the language code and predominantly receptive aphasia is primarily a disorder of language decoding. Fourth, aphasia as a language disorder, affects cognitive and psychological processing of verbal symbols. Fifth, because of the multitude of associated related symptoms and characteristics, aphasia is a syndrome.

Understanding Aphasia Diagnostic Terminology

As discussed in Chapter 2, there are many classification systems of aphasia and each reflects a theory about the nature of this neurogenic communication disorder. This has led to controversy about the characteristic to which each aphasia diagnostic term refers. Table 3.1 shows three general classification categories, the assumed primary site of brain and central nervous system damage, and conventional terminology for specific aphasia diagnostic labels. The neuroanatomical reference sites of lesions are Broca and Wernicke's areas and/or the tracts of the brain leading to and from them.

Table 3.1: Aphasia Diagnostic Terminology

Damage to Broca's and/or Adjacent Areas/Tracts of the Brain	Damage to Wernicke's and/or Adjacent Areas/Tracts of the Brain	Damage to Broca's, Wernicke's, and/or Adjacent Areas/Tracts of the Brain
Broca's aphasia	Wernicke's aphasia	Global Aphasia
Predominantly expressive aphasia	Predominantly receptive aphasia	Severe expressive-receptive aphasia
Motor aphasia	Sensory aphasia	Dense aphasia
Nonfluent aphasia	Fluent jargon aphasia	Irreversible aphasia syndrome
Anterior aphasia	Posterior aphasia	Anterior-posterior, mixed aphasia

In the early 1900s, Korbinian Brodmann, a German neurologist, created the brain mapping system that bears his name. He identified 52 functional sites of the brain based on their stained visual appearance. Later, some of the original sites were further subdivided to more clearly reflect their location and function. Broca's area is located in

Brodmann Area 44, the inferior frontal gyrus of the left cerebral hemisphere. Most authorities also include Brodmann Area 45, the pars triangularis of the inferior frontal gyrus, as part of Broca's area. Wernicke's area is located in Brodmann Areas 22, 41, and 42 (Kent, 1997) in the superior part of the left temporal lobe which is also known as the superior temporal area and the primary auditory cortex. Some authorities extend Wernicke's area into the parietal lobe and include Brodmann area 39 and Brodmann area 40, the angular and supramarginal sections, which are involved in reading and alexia. The diagnostic labels of *Broca* and *Wernicke's aphasia* refer to damage to the above areas and/or the tracts leading to and from them. When both areas are damaged, the neurogenic communication disorder is labeled *global aphasia*. Figure 3.1 shows approximate sites of major speech and hearing landmarks of the brain.

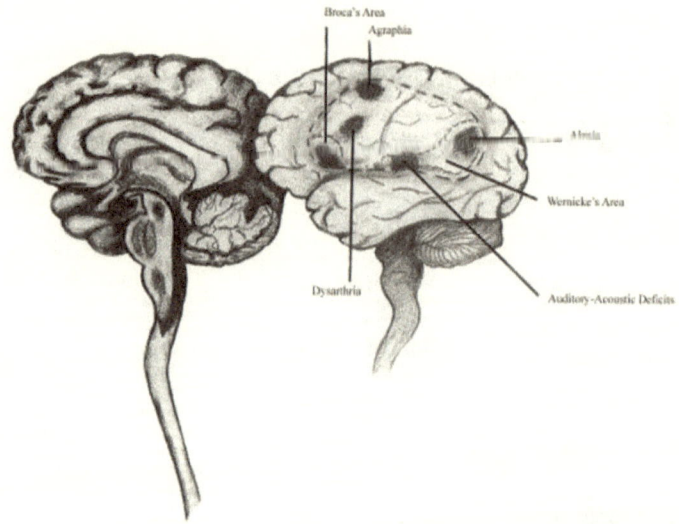

Figure 3.1: Approximate boundaries of expressive and receptive speech and language centers

The diagnostic labels *predominantly expressive aphasia* and *predominantly receptive aphasia* suggest that aphasia cuts across all modalities of expression and reception. In predominantly expressive aphasia, the primary communication disorders involve speaking, writing, and using expressive gestures. In predominantly receptive aphasia, the primary communication disorders involve reading, and understanding the speech and gestures of others. In many cases, it may appear that only language expression or reception is impaired, however, detailed testing will show that the aphasia, more or less, cuts across all language modalities. Corresponding to global aphasia is *severe expressive-receptive aphasia* with major disruptions in both expressive and receptive language functions.

In the current view of neurogenic communication disorders, motor aphasia is an oxymoron. Because aphasia is a language disorder and not a speech pathology, motor aphasia is a contradiction in diagnostic terms. However, some authorities on aphasia use the motor-sensory aphasia distinction. *Motor aphasia*, an expressive disorder, results from damage to Broca's area and/or adjacent areas and tracts of the brain. *Sensory aphasia*, a receptive disorder, results from damage to Wernicke's area and/or adjacent areas and tracts of the brain. Extensive damage to both areas is sometimes called *dense aphasia* referring to a large mass of brain and central nervous system damage.

In nonfluent-fluent aphasia diagnostic terminology, the patient's speech and language fluency distinguishes expressive and receptive impairments. *Nonfluent aphasia*, an expressive aphasia, includes decreased output overall, effort and struggle to produce speech, decreased phrase length, and prosodic disturbances. Motor speech disorders are often present in nonfluent aphasia. *Fluent aphasia,* a receptive aphasia, is associated with reduced auditory and reading comprehension and the expressive component is sometimes referred to as *fluent jargon aphasia.* Fluent aphasia speakers produce speech with little effort and struggle, and with normal prosody, but the output is semantically inappropriate. The structure of fluent aphasia appears normal, but the content is without meaning. "Thus, although they speak at a quite normal speaking rate, sounds shift and words blend in their speech. Sometimes whole utterances consist of neologisms, nonexisting words that sound like but are not words of the speaker's language" (Laakso, 2003, p. 163). Severe damage to the important speech and language centers of the brain is considered irreversible.

In the anterior and posterior aphasia distinction, the dividing neuroanatomical line is the fissure of Rolando also called the central sulcus. The fissure of Rolando separates the frontal and parietal lobes. *Anterior aphasia* is nonfluent and agrammatic. Patients with anterior aphasia have problems writing, using expressive gestures, and repeating. *Posterior aphasia* is fluent and meaningless. Patients with posterior aphasia have problems reading and understanding the speech and complicated gestures of others. Damage to both regions is *mixed* or *anterior-posterior aphasia.*

Other diagnostic terms for aphasia generally refer to the patient's impaired ability to retrieve words in conversational speech and during confrontational naming tasks. When alternate words are used for the desired one, there is usually rhyme or reason relationship to them. In *literal paraphasia*, the alternate word phonemically resembles the desired one, e.g., gun, fun. In *verbal paraphasia*, there is a semantic relationship, e.g., pen, pencil (See Chapter 2). In *random neologistic paraphasias*, there appears to be no phonemic or semantic relationship between the alternate word and the desired one.

> "In conversation with aphasic persons, collaboration of the non-aphasic participants is needed in order for the conversation to succeed" (Laakso, 2003, p. 180).

Language Encoding Disorders

Language encoding is formulating and transforming cognitive information into an expressive linguistic code. It is the process by which humans express thoughts through speaking, writing, and expressive gestures. As Table 3.1 shows, the expressive aphasia disorders go by several diagnostic labels including Broca's, predominantly expressive, motor, nonfluent, and anterior aphasia. Clinically, the *verbal encoding disorder* is characterized by wordfinding problems, a language disorder, and verbal apraxia, a motor speech programming deficit. *Agraphia* is the expressive encoding disorder affecting writing. The expressive encoding disorder affecting the ability to engage in complicated gestures for communication purposes is referred to as *Aphasic Expressive Gestural Involvement* (AEGI).

Aphasic Verbal Encoding Disorder

Two clinical features characterize the *Aphasic Verbal Encoding Disorder* (AVED) verbal output seen in Broca's, predominantly expressive, motor, nonfluent, anterior aphasia: *wordfinding impairments* and *verbal apraxia*. Wordfinding impairments, problems recalling words for expression, occur during confrontation naming tasks and conversational speech. Verbal apraxia, also called apraxia of speech, is impairment of the ability to conceptualize, program, and execute voluntary neuromuscular speech movements. Although each clinical feature may occur independently, both usually occur together in classic aphasias such as those resulting from cerebral vascular accidents. Typically, aphasic patients with the verbal encoding disorders can be divided into those with a *preponderance* of wordfinding impairments and those with primarily verbal apraxia symptoms. Patients with a preponderance of wordfinding impairments essentially have problems with recalling words for verbal expression while those with a predominance of verbal apraxia primarily have more difficulty motorically uttering recalled words.

Wordfinding Impairments

Wordfinding impairments are problems aphasic patients have recalling words to express themselves verbally. Although several diagnostic terms can be used to label this language disorder such as semantic aphasia, anomia, nominal aphasia, naming deficits, and amnestic aphasia, these terms often have vague and sometimes disparate clinical definitions. Some terms refer to a general category of aphasia or the verbal output seen in some patients with traumatic brain injuries, psychiatric conditions, and dementia. There are seven types of wordfinding behaviors in aphasic patients: *mutism, literal phonemic approximations, verbal semantic associations, delay, description, generalization,* and *tip-of-the-tongue* behaviors.

During conversational speech or during confrontation naming exercises, some aphasic patients are mute. When wanting to recall a word during conversation or confronted with the task of labeling or naming something or someone, they cannot conjure any verbal response and are mute overall or for the particular task. They are wordless to express the particular referent or concept.

As discussed above, literal phonemic approximation paraphasias occur when the aphasic patient produces a phonemically similar but erroneous word for the desired one. The aphasic patient may say "fell" for "smell," "fun" for "run," or "kun" for "gun." While there are similarities between the struggled attempt to produce a word occurring in verbal apraxia and literal phonemic approximation paraphasias, the latter are phonologically-based and not exclusively a motor programming disorder.

Some aphasic patients may produce verbal semantic association paraphasias during wordfinding behaviors. Verbal semantic association paraphasias occur when the aphasic patient produces a semantically related word for the appropriate one. It is an inaccurate circumlocution such as uttering "car" for "truck," "hand" for "foot," or "chair" for "table."

Marshall (1976, p. 446), in a classic study on word retrieval behavior of aphasic adults, identified three additional varieties of wordfinding behaviors: *delay, description,* and *generalization:*

> Delay: The patient takes or requests additional time to produce the word. Although some delay is certainly inherent in all retrieval efforts, in this case subjects tended to use a filled pause, unfilled pause or some stalling tactic to let the listener know they did not want to be interrupted and needed more time to produce the word.

> Description: Subjects attempted to produce the desired word by describing what they were talking about. Although associational behaviors were often observed within the context of subjects' descriptions, the examples

. . . clearly indicate the necessity on the part of the patient to tell something about the intended word.

Generalization: Here subjects produced general words . . . in place of the desired word. In many instances, this behavior seemed to represent a manipulative effort on part of the aphasic to get the clinician to supply the needed word.

The tip-of-the-tongue phenomenon is what occurs when the patient engages in phonemic and semantic trial-and-error behaviors to find the desired and correct word. In this frustrating behavior, the word appears just out of reach and the patient makes repetitive attempts to say it. The tip-of-the-tongue phenomenon is part of the wordfinding and motor speech production deficits.

Verbal Apraxia

Once the word has been recalled, some patients with Broca's, predominantly expressive, motor, nonfluent, anterior aphasia have difficulty programming it into existence. The patient has the word in his or her internal monologue, he or she has recalled it in inner speech, but programming the neuromuscular actions necessary to produce it is impaired or nonexistent.

Verbal apraxia, a motor speech disorder, is examined in detail in Chapter 5. Verbal apraxia refers to the impaired ability to conceptualize, program, and execute voluntary neuromuscular speech movements. Verbal apraxia primarily affects articulation, but can impair, more or less, other motor speech processes such as respiration, phonation, and resonance. A key aspect of verbal apraxia is *automatic speech.* Although purposeful and volitional utterances are difficult or impossible to produce, many patients have automatic speech which is sometimes called *subcortical speech.* When little thought and attention are given to the utterance, some patients can say over-learned and automatic utterances such as swear words, names of family members, and rote-learned phrases. Patients with Broca's, predominantly expressive, motor, nonfluent, anterior aphasia with a predominance of verbal apraxia have more difficulty voluntarily programming words into existence than recalling them for expression.

In verbal encoding disorders, the output of the aphasic patient is influenced by his or her *awareness of errors* and the ability to *self-correct*. A patient with awareness of errors knows when he or she has recalled the desired word and produced it correctly. The patient who is self-corrective, through trial and error, can eventually recall and correctly produce the desired word.

The following is an example of the Aphasic Verbal Encoding Disorder (AVED) (Tanner, 2007a, p. 72):

> I, swant, uh, want, to say, play, choker; not choker, uh, (pause) choker. No. Poker. I want to say poker today, uh, tonight, with my daught . . . , strife, uh strife, uh, (pause) wife. I bet quarter. Straw choker, uh, uh, foker, uh, forker, forker, puh, orker is game. Damn it, draw poker is my game,

In the above example, the patient displays wordfinding impairments on the words "poker," "today," "wife," and "draw." Verbal apraxia is present on "want," "poker," "wife," and "draw." "Damn it, draw poker is my game" is an example of automatic speech. For the most part, the patient is aware of errors and usually self-corrective.

Verbal apraxia is often seen initially in brain injuries, the but because of the reduction of brain edema and other factors, it often subsides or disappears completely.

Aphasic Agraphia

All normal children are born with the ability to speak using verbal symbols, but humans must be taught to write. Formulating and transforming cognitive information into a written linguistic code is a learned behavior. Written expression shares the essential elements of verbal expression in that it is an arbitrary symbolic representation of reality and rule-dependent.

Aphasic agraphia (AA) is an acquired inability to express oneself in writing not due to arm and hand paralysis. While it is true that many patients with Broca's, predominantly expressive, motor, nonfluent, anterior aphasia may have weak or nonfunctional arms and hands, their core writing problems are not due to paralysis. To illustrate that aphasic agraphia is a disorder of graphic symbolism and not fundamentally a motor problem, patients with severe aphasia cannot meaningfully express themselves in writing even when they hold the pen or pencil in their non-paralyzed hand. Most persons can write with their non-dominant hands, albeit with less legibility.

With few exceptions, aphasic patients write like they speak. Patients with fluent jargon write using meaningless written signs, letters, words, and phrases. Nonfluent patients write haltingly, with many errors of letter form; words are typically misspelled and writing is a perplexing struggle. Because aphasic agraphia is a central graphic language processing disorder, spelling impairments usually accompanies it. Pelagie and Hillis (2001, p. 590) emphasize the critical role spelling impairments play in agraphia: "Spelling impairments can result from damage to one or more of the critical components of the cognitive processes that support written spelling."

Pelagie and Hillis (2001) list four types of acquired agraphia: *deep, surface, global,* and *graphemic buffer.* Deep agraphia is a problem with written semantic errors and poor phoneme-to-grapheme conversion. Surface agraphia results in partial knowledge of written word forms: "In many cases of acquired agraphia, patients appear to have lost the graphemic representations for words, or have degraded representations, so that they show partial knowledge of word forms that they once knew" (Pelagie and Hillis, 2001, p. 586). Global agraphia is a writing impairment characterized by a limited number of correctly spelled high frequency words and a complete inability to spell nonwords. Graphemic buffer agraphia is a decay of short term writing memory so that information about the identity and serial ordering of letters is disrupted. The result is grapheme omissions, substitutions, transpositions, and additions. Benson and Ardila (1996) list "pure agraphia" as likely occurring as a result of damage to the left premotor cortex. Rosati and DeBastiani (1979) consider pure agraphia to be a separate and distinct form of aphasia.

Aphasic Expressive Gestural Involvement

There are two general types of *Aphasic Expressive Gestural Involvement* (AEGI) impairments that accompany verbal communication: *descriptive* and *reinforcing gestural disorders.* A descriptive gesture, as the name implies, involves the speaker using facial, arm, and hand gestures to provide direction or explain an action. Expressive reinforcing gestures are used to emphasize, accentuate, and stress a verbal statement sending information about how the person feels. Expressive gestural communication ranges from simple body movements showing escape and avoidance to complex, language-based gestures involving finger-spelling and sign language. According to Davis (2007), gestures can be evaluated with regard to the *transivity* and *complexity* of body movements. An example of a transitive action on an object is dialing the telephone and an intransitive action without an object is displaying the "thumbs up" sign. The complexity of gestural expression ranges from single movements such as pantomiming the drinking of water from a glass to sequenced gestures such as showing the steps necessary to get out of bed and go to the bathroom. Kearns and Elman (2001) also include *role playing* and *psychodrama* to act out emotions associated with aphasia as sophisticated gestural communication.

In 1963, Goodglass and Kaplan reported in the neurology journal *Brain* that aphasia impairs the ability to communicate ideas through gesture and pantomime. However, many previous theorists and researchers, especially those noting that this language disorder impairs all modalities of communication (See Chapter 2), also reported the idea-gesture disconnect in aphasia. Most aphasic patients can express pain, avoidance, escape, and some simple wants and needs through primitive gestures and reactive body movements. Never-the-less, expressing thoughts through elaborate signs and complex pantomime is beyond the capabilities of most patients with this acquired language disorder. Patients with Broca's, predominantly expressive, motor, nonfluent, anterior aphasia have various degrees of impairments expressing themselves using gestures and pantomime for expressive purposes. Patients with pure motor speech disorders are more likely to be successful using elaborate signs, communication boards, and complex pantomime to express themselves. However, even for patients with pure motor speech disorders, *limb apraxia*, the inability to engage in purposeful complex body movements, impairs functional gestural expression.

> Kinetics is the study of body movements including the use of gestures during speech communication.

Language Decoding Disorders

Language decoding is converting expressed language into an understandable linguistic code and processing the information cognitively. It is the process by which humans comprehend and understand the thoughts expressed through speaking, writing, and expressive gestures. As Table 3.1 shows, receptive aphasia disorders go by several diagnostic labels including Wernicke's, predominantly receptive, sensory, fluent, and posterior aphasia. *Aphasic Verbal Decoding Disorder (AVDD)* is the inability auditorially to comprehend spoken language and *alexia* is the inability to decode written information. The receptive decoding disorder affecting the ability to understand complicated gestures and pantomime is referred to as *receptive gestural involvement*.

Aphasic Verbal Decoding Disorder

The *aphasic verbal decoding disorder* (AVDD) is primarily a disorder of semantics. Patients with this type of neurogenic communication disorder have an inability or reduced ability to comprehend spoken language. In addition, most patients with this predominantly receptive disorder also have fundamental disruptions in the ability verbally to express themselves. This expressive component is called *fluent jargon aphasia.*

Auditory Comprehension Disorders

Auditory comprehension of spoken language is dependent on the sense of hearing and auditory perception. As discussed in Chapter 4, the structures of the hearing mechanism transform the acoustic energy generated by the speaker into mechanical, hydraulic, and electrochemical energy. Auditory neural impulses are routed through cranial nerve VIII to the thalamus where the first stage of perception occurs. At the level of the thalamus, basal meaning is attached to auditory sensation and the perceived salient information is gated to Wernicke's and other areas of the brain. Higher level decoding of the perceived auditory information involves extracting the denotative and connotative meaning from individual words, sentences, phrases, and discourse.

In a trend that began in the 1800s with Karl Wernicke's identification of the "sensory" or "receptive" language sites of the left temporal lobe, modern textbooks continue to attribute this area as the "center for language understanding." In Lee Edward Travis' classic textbook, *Handbook for Speech Pathology and Audiology,* Wood (1971, p. 23) defines Wernicke's area as "a region in the superior convolution of the temporal lobe of the cerebrum identified as the center for understanding speech heard." *Stedman's Concise Medical Dictionary for the Health Professions* (4th ed.) defines Wernicke's area as: "The region of the cerebral cortex thought to be essential for understanding and formulating coherent, propositional speech . . . " (Dirckx, 2001, p. 1066). Nicolosi, Harryman, and Kresheck (2004, p. 343) in *Terminology of Communication Disorders: Speech-Language-Hearing* (5th ed.) define Wernicke's area as: "Region in the superior convolution of the temporal lobe of the cerebrum which is identified as the center for understanding oral language; corresponds approximately to Brodmann's areas 22, 39, and 40."

While Wernicke's area may be an important cortical conduit for decoding sensory, perceptual, phonological, grammatical, and semantic features of oral language, attributing this site as the "center for oral language understanding" is based on inexact and narrow definitions of the words "understand," "comprehend," and "center." Oxford Dictionary (2005) defines "understand" as the perception of the meaning of words, appreciation of the significance of a statement, interpretation of the implications of an idea, and inferences that can be drawn from a statement. *Webster's New World College Dictionary* (2000) makes the distinction that while "understand" and "comprehend" are used interchangeably, the former stresses the full awareness or knowledge arrived at. The word "center," Greek for *kentron* or "sharp point," typically means "primary," "core," and "principal."

There is no one "center" for language "understanding and comprehension" for these are sophisticated, complicated cognitive functions that engage widespread cortical and subcortical areas of the brain. Perhaps more than any other language function, the process of auditory understanding and comprehension involves the brain operating as a whole and the totality of the mind. "To propose that Wernicke's area of the brain, this small mass of brain cells and the tracts leading to and from it, is the "center" for verbal "understanding" . . . is inexact and inaccurate" (Tanner, 2007b, p. X). Consequently, damage to Wernicke's area of the brain affects decoding of sensory, perceptual, phonological, grammatical, and semantic features of language, but only in the context of a cortical conduit to the larger processes of oral language understanding and comprehension.

Patients with aphasic verbal decoding impairments have auditory comprehension deficits not attributable to hearing loss, deafness, and the modality specific perceptual disorders of auditory or acoustic agnosia. However, because of the verbal decoding dependency on the auditory sensory and perceptual systems, it is necessary briefly to review their roles in the process. Before verbal decoding can occur, there must be *general auditory perception* involving sound detection, localization, and identification. Prior to verbal decoding, the listener detects sound emanating from the speaker and selectively attends to it. The signal is categorized as speech, separate and distinct from all other environmental sounds. The sound is localized in space and time, and there is gross identification of vowels and consonants to determine the nature of the sound and language being spoken.

Speech discrimination, a combination of auditory sensation and basal perception, involves the analysis of speech acoustics and the distinctive features of the speech signal. Based on past auditory perceptual experiences, the listener analyzes the acoustic characteristics of each phoneme, i.e., acoustic patterns of time, frequency, energy, and their distinctive features, and compares them in auditory memory. Patients with impairments of general auditory perception and speech discrimination have auditory sensation and perceptual disorders which impair or prevent higher level speech signal decoding.

Verbal decoding of the above auditory sensation and basal perceptual information begins with semantic extraction of the denotative meanings of words and associated grammatical constructs. Denotative meanings of words are their explicit primary meanings. At this level, the listener associates the individual words with his or her previous experiences and evokes the lexical and dictionary meanings of them. At the denotative extraction level, which is the fundamental symbol-referent relationship of semantics, the verbal symbol and its referent are associated. Semantic meaning lies in the relationship between the word and that to which it represents. For tangible and concrete words, there is usually a visual image of the referent. For intangible and more abstract words, the process involves verbal associations. For example, extracting the denotative meaning of "chair" involves its visual icon while extracting the denotative meaning of "truth" involves verbally associating the lexical and dictionary definitions of the word.

Decoding the connotations of words is making personal and logical associations about them. Connotation semantics are implied meanings of words and associated grammatical constructs, including their lexical and dictionary definitions, and also the personal emotive reactions logically implied by them. For example, the connotation of the word "teacher" may include what is denoted by the word, i.e., someone who imparts information, but also the emotive reactions logically implied and suggested: a particular person, an individual with specialized knowledge, a mentor, a disciplinarian, and so forth.

Dynamic symbolism is the highest and most comprehensive level of verbal decoding Tanner (2007b). Dynamic symbolism is based on the philosophy of General Semantics advanced by Alfred Korzybski, a Polish mathematician and engineer in the early 1900s. In General Semantics, the statement, "The map is not the territory" illustrates the highly variable relationship between the word, the map, to its meaning, the territory. General Semantics takes a non-Aristotelian relativistic view of humans as time-binding semantic reactors. According to General Semantics, the meanings of words are relative and a result of accumulated and ongoing personal and social experiences. General Semantics refers to itself as "up-to-date, applied epistemology" and bases its philosophy on the scientific method (Institute of General Semantics, 2007). General Semantics attempts to make a person continuously aware of the process of verbal abstraction.

Dynamic symbolism is the process of assimilating abstract words, and ongoing integrating of their meanings into the decoder's frame-of-reference. In dynamic symbolism, not only are new symbol-referent associations made, but previous connections are continuously modified to account for changes in word meanings occurring overtime. Auditory comprehension is an ongoing process of receiving environmental information and continuously adjusting the parameters of what is to be perceived and associated. Various labels have been given to aphasic verbal decoding disorders involving the extraction of semantic meaning including anomia, amnesic, amnestic, nominal, and semantic aphasias.

Fluent Jargon

Fluent jargon occurs in many patients with the aphasic verbal encoding disorder. Fluent jargon is described as verbalization without semantic substance and is sometimes labeled "word salad" and "logorrhea." In fluent jargon, prosody, rate, rhythm, intonation, stress, and cadence of speech are normal, but the output is semantically impaired or completely lacking in meaningful content. The fluent jargon aphasic patient's output consists of literal phonemic approximation paraphasias, an alternate word phonemically resembling the desired one, verbal semantic association paraphasias, substitutions with a semantic relationship, and random neologistic paraphasias, where there is no apparent phonemic or semantic relationship between the substituted and appropriate word. Fluent jargon aphasic patients usually exhibit a preponderance of paraphasia types; some patients produce predominantly verbal semantic associations, others produce predominantly literal phonemic approximations, and others primarily random neologistic paraphasias.

The primary site of lesion in fluent jargon patients is Wernicke's area of the left dominant hemisphere of the brain. Cappa, Cavallotti, and Vignolo (1981) found that patients displaying a predominance of verbal semantic association paraphasias have primary damage to the posterior angular gyrus and adjacent areas while those patients producing *predominantly literal phonemic approximation paraphasia* have primary damage to Wernicke's area extending into the inferior parietal lobe. On a perceptual-cognitive continuum level, it is likely that patients producing predominantly literal phonemic approximation paraphasia have auditory comprehension disorders primarily at the perceptual level. Patients with predominantly verbal semantic association paraphasias have higher level verbal association errors.

Correlating the phonemic and lexical errors in aphasia with the lesion sites may shed light on the neurophysiology of language in general and fluent jargon in particular, but it does not explain why patients with so-called "receptive" aphasia have dramatically impaired verbal expression. To complicate the issue, the fluent jargon seen in aphasia is similar, if not identical, to the verbal output in schizophrenic language (Benson and Ardila, 1996; Chaika, 1974, and others). While there is no general agreement among scientists and clinicians, there are four possible reasons why many patients with damage to Wernicke's and adjacent areas of the brain have fluent jargon.

The first reason patients with predominantly receptive aphasia speak with meaningless fluent jargon is because the receptive-expressive language dichotomy is artificial and not based on functional brain neuroanatomy and physiology. This is particularly true when motor speech disorders are considered distinct and separate from the language disorder of aphasia. Brownell (2000) notes that expressive and receptive vocabularies are similar, but expressive vocabulary requires access to the words for memory retrieval and production. Zimmerman, Steiner, and Pond (1992, p. 5) consider receptive and expressive language fundamentally related in cognitive development:

> It is generally assumed that receptive and expressive skills are related, with receptive acquisition of a language skill serving, in most cases, as a precursor to the expressive acquisition of that skill. A child must learn to recognize a word that he or she hears others use for an object. The child must also learn to associate the word with the object before he or she can produce the word for the object.

Zimmerman, Steiner, and Pond (1992) note that receptive knowledge is not perfect before expressive use begins; the child may only have a general idea of what a referent is before using the word to refer to it.

Second, fluent jargon may result from the patient being unable to monitor his or her output; it is meaningless because of poor self-monitoring. Because of the auditory comprehension disorder, the patient cannot understand his or her own speech any better than the speech of others. The fluent jargon patient does not know when nonsense is being uttered so he or she continues to speak as if the output is meaningful.

The third reason for fluent jargon occurring in patients with "receptive" aphasia concerns the *language-thought controversy*. The language-thought controversy is whether language simply expresses thought or if it is a fundamental aspect of thinking. If language is the former, then the fluent jargon patient has normal *internal monologues*, inner speech, and is simply expressing his or her thoughts abnormally. This is unlikely and assumes that internal verbal thoughts are not affected by brain damage that impairs externalized language. Critchley (1970), and others, note that aphasia impairs general verbal symbolism. Current research using modern brain scanning instruments show that brain injury does not disrupt externalized language while preserving inner speech linguistic codes. The fluent jargon patient's expressed thoughts are the same as his or her internal monologues; he or she is expressing mixed-up ideas. In addition, the fluent jargon patient's non-language cognition is relatively intact and, as Darley (1982) notes, language code processing impairments in aphasia are disproportionate to dysfunctions in other cognitive areas. The patient's general semantic processing is damaged for verbal expression, auditory association, and inner speech. However, this is not to say that the fluent jargon patient's thoughts and expressions do not have meaning to him or her in a psychological sense.

The fourth reason for fluent jargon in receptive aphasia concerns psychological defense mechanisms and coping styles. Many patients with fluent jargon engage in *denial-projection* about their communication disorders. If not for the psychological defenses and coping styles of denial and projection, the fluent jargon in aphasic patients would be short-lived. Many fluent jargon patients persist in making meaningless utterances even though it is apparent that no substantial communication occurs with doctors, nurses, therapists, and family members. These patients deny their communication disorders and project them to listeners. Because of denial and projection, they act as though meaningful communication would occur if others would simply try harder to understand their "perfectly normal" utterances. Weinstein and Puig-Antich (1974) and Weinstein, Lyerly, Cole, and Ozer (1966) address meaning and denial in fluent jargon aphasia in the journal *Cortex*.

> The denial and lack of awareness seen in jargon aphasia is a deterrent to therapy. A patient must be aware of his or her disability to overcome it.

The following is an example of fluent jargon in a male patient answering the question: How are you doing?

"The acrylic thus far is preponderance. Tula, est tula, and the acrylic must be made. I am acrylic thus far. Don't you know. (Laughter). Of course, the preponderance of the acrylic is chet jitters and acrylic thus far. So much for that."

In the above example of jargon aphasia, the patient understood that the question concerns his medical condition. The phonemic jargon words, speech sounds combined which do not make sense, are "tula," "est tula," "chet" and "jitters." Semantic jargon, use of conventional words in meaningless context involved "acrylic," "preponderance," and "thus far." He also laughed because the listener was unable to understand his "perfectly normal" speech.

Aphasic Alexia

Dyslexia is a type of reading problem seen in school children which is substantially different from the reading problems in adult neurogenic communication disorders. Dyslexia is a learning disability and essentially a visual perceptual disorder where letters are juxtaposed, reversed, or inverted. Shaywitz and Shaywitz (2007) note that dyslexia in children involves a failure of the left-hemisphere posterior brain systems, particularly the left occipito-temporal region, to function normally. *Aphasic alexia* in adults with neurogenic communication disorders can include the above perceptual impairments, but it is primarily a loss of written word meanings. Beeson and Hillis (2001) note that reading is dependent on visual analysis of letter strings, graphemic input vocabulary, and letter-to-sound conversion. The primary distinguishing features between dyslexia and aphasic alexia are perceptual and associational impairments. Beeson and Hillis

(2001, p. 573) comment on semantic processing and reading: "For example, semantic processing is necessary for auditory comprehension tasks, writing, and oral naming, as well as reading. Similarly, the phonological output lexicon is assessed for both oral naming and oral reading tasks."

Unfortunately, some authorities also use the label "word blindness" to refer to the reading problems seen in patients with neurogenic communication disorders suggesting that the core problem is with eye-blindness. Although strokes, head traumas, and diseases that cause neurogenic communication disorders can cause blindness and visual fields deficits, the reading disorder of aphasic alexia is not a result of the patient having problems seeing the printed or handwritten word. However, *homonymous hemianopsia* is a type of visual field deficiency and blindness occurring in neurogenic communication disorders. It is the loss of the same visual half-field of both eyes. Patients are said to have right or left homonymous hemianopsia to refer to blindness in either the right or left fields of both eyes. Additionally, these patients usually have *visual neglect,* the lack of awareness of stimuli on the affected side of their bodies.

While patients with aphasic alexia may have co-occurring eye-blindness, homonymous hemianopsia, tunnel vision, and other visual sensory and perceptual deficits, this language decoding disorder is fundamentally a problem semantically decoding written words. Aphasic alexia is a central graphic decoding disorder. Aphasic *alexia with agraphia* is sometimes referred to as parietal agraphia (Roeltgin, 1993). Some authorities distinguish between *surface* and *deep* (dyslexia) *alexia* (Marshall and Newcombe (1973, 1966). Surface alexia is a problem "sounding out" written graphemes. Deep alexia involves the patient producing semantic associations when reading aloud. A patient with deep alexia interprets the written word through his or her disordered semantic processor and reads, not the word, but what he or she "thinks" it says, thus producing verbal semantic association paraphasias. Other factors may also be involved in aphasic alexia. The patient may have reduced attention and have difficulty grasping the entire idea of a text. There is a rare reading disorder in neurogenic communication disorders called *alexia without agraphia*. With this disorder, the patient has trouble reading, but writing is done relatively well. Remarkably, some patients with alexia without agraphia cannot read what they have just written.

Aphasic Receptive Gestural Involvement

The aphasic gestural communication problem discussed in the section on language encoding disorders is not limited to the patient's inability to express himself or herself through gesture and pantomime; it is also a gestural understanding and comprehension disorder. Understanding and comprehending gestures range from grasping the intent of simple one-movement hand actions, such as beckoning someone using the index finger, to making sense of complex pantomimes and appreciating the nuances of interpretative dance. It also includes appreciating the nonverbal effects of facial expression. This impairment is referred to as *aphasic receptive gestural involvement*.

Impairment of understanding and comprehending gestural communication in aphasic patients is associated with other language-based disorders. Duffy, Duffy, and Pearson (1975) found that aphasic naming deficits, auditory comprehension disorders, and general language impairments correlate with impaired pantomime recognition. Varney (1978) looked at the linguistic correlates of pantomime recognition in aphasic patients and reports a strong relationship between reading and *pantomime comprehension disorders*.

Understanding and comprehending gestures, particularly regarding nonverbal communication and emotion, and the interpretation of visual-spatial-temporal physical actions, involve the right hemisphere of the brain. "The concept that the right hemisphere processes (i.e., recognizes and expresses) emotional phenomena appears to be generally accepted" (Sarno and Gainotti, 1998, p. 573). However, the idea that the right hemisphere of the brain has entirely different functions with regard to interpreting emotions and gestures is misleading. According to Bruer (1999), the facts do not support claims about the generally accepted belief that the two hemispheres of the brain have vastly different functions; both hemispheres are involved in almost every processing task.

Cortical representation of prepositions provides a good example of bi-hemispheric and visual-spatial-temporal brain functions. Conventional brain-based learning models and linguistic localization theories postulate language as a left-hemisphere phenomenon in most persons. However, with just a moment's thought, it must be recognized that prepositional concepts such as "in," "beside," "below," "above," and so forth are as much visual-spatial-temporal concepts as linguistic ones. The same is true for interpreting gestures as linguistic symbols. Table 3.2 classifies and summarizes the encoding and decoding in aphasia.

Table 3.2: Aphasia--A Language Encoding and Decoding Disorder

Language Function	Symptoms and Manifestations
Language Encoding Impairments	Aphasic Verbal Encoding Disorder (AVED)
	-Wordfinding Impairments
	-Verbal Apraxia
	Aphasic Agraphia (AA)
	Aphasic Expressive Gesture Involvement (AEGI)
Language Decoding Impairments	Aphasic Verbal Decoding Disorder (AVDD)
	-Auditory Comprehension Disorders
	-Fluent Jargon
	Aphasic Alexia (AA)
	Aphasic Receptive Gestural Involvement (ARGI)

Transcortical and Conduction Aphasias

The patient's ability to repeat is the defining characteristic in *transcortical motor, conduction,* and *transcortical sensory* aphasias (See Table 3.3). Localizationists consider these disorders "disconnect aphasias" resulting from damage to association tracts which connect one cortical region to another (Davis, 2007). The failure of a patient to repeat what has been spoken by others can be caused by several neurological and cognitive defects, but damage to the fibers and tracts connecting Wernicke's and Broca's areas is considered the primary site of lesion in disconnect aphasias. For the most part, the lesion's proximity to Wernicke's or Broca's areas affect the type of symptoms seen in transcortical and conduction aphasias.

Transcortical motor aphasia can be considered a manifestation of the verbal encoding disorder of Broca's, predominantly expressive, motor, nonfluent, anterior aphasia. According to Damiaso (1998), patients with transcortical motor aphasia have the ability to repeat, impaired auditory comprehension when tested formally, and *echolalia*, the echoing and automatic repetition of what has been spoken by another person. Transcortical motor aphasia results from damage to various sites in the frontal lobe and resembles Broca's aphasia but with preserved repetition (Davis, 2007).

"The speech of conduction aphasics is fluent although usually less abundant than that of Wernicke's. Commonly there are minor defects in aural comprehension, although understanding of colloquial conversation is intact" (Damiaso, 1998, p. 35). Davis (2007) suggests the key symptom in conduction aphasia is "surprisingly" impaired repetition. Damage to subcortical white matter structures and association tracts, particularly the *arcuate fasciculus*, have been identified as sites of lesions in conduction aphasia.

Transcortical sensory aphasia can be considered a manifestation of the verbal decoding disorder of Wernicke's, predominantly receptive, sensory, fluent, and posterior aphasia. Patients with transcortical sensory aphasia have preserved repetition yet severely impaired auditory comprehension and fluent, paraphasic speech (Damiaso, 1998). According to Davis (2007), the likely site of lesion in transcortical sensory aphasia is the temporo-occipital border or the area between the middle and posterior cerebral arteries.

Table 3.3: Transcortical and Conduction Aphasias

Type of Aphasia	Approximate Site of Brain Lesion	Effects on Patient's Ability to Repeat Spoken Language
Transcortical Motor Aphasia	Various Sites in the Frontal Lobe	Patient Can Repeat Words Spoken by Others
Conduction Aphasia	Damage to Subcortical White Matter Structures and Association Tracts (Arcuate Fasciculus)	Impaired Repetition
Transcortical Sensory Aphasia	Temporo-Occipital Border or the Area Between the Middle and Posterior Cerebral Arteries	Patient Can Repeat Words Spoken by Others

The requirement of making diagnostic distinctions with regard to transcortical motor, transcortical sensory, and conduction aphasia is a remnant of pre-modern clinical brain scanning technology. In the past, neurologists diagnosed the site of lesion in aphasia based on detailed analysis of the patient's language and motor speech impairments. The patient's ability or inability to repeat utterances spoken by others, and co-occurring with other aphasic symptoms, provided neurologists with valuable information about the site of lesion and the nature of the brain damage. However, modern brain scanning devices are available which have eliminated the need to diagnose site of lesion by detailed analysis of aphasic symptoms. Today, knowledge of whether a patient can or cannot repeat utterances spoken by others is simply one evaluative and treatment factor in a patient's comprehensive profile of symptoms. While transcortical and conduction aphasias are neurologically interesting to study, and shed light on human neurology in general, designating separate categories of aphasia based on the patient's ability to engage in repetition is an artifact of past neurological diagnostic practices. Because of modern brain scanning technology, the presence or absence of the ability to repeat is no more clinically remarkable than the myriad of other aphasic manifestations.

Subcortical, Progressive, and Atypical Aphasias

The existence of *subcortical aphasias* is controversial and dependent on the definition of language. Subcortical aphasias occur because of damage to brain structures below the cortex in the language dominant hemisphere. According to Benson and Ardila (1996), this area is known as Marie's quadrilateral space which includes the *caudate nucleus, putamen, internal capsule,* and *thalamus.* However, particularly in multiple infarct strokes and diffuse traumatic brain injuries, the distinction between isolated cortical and subcortical brain damage is vague. In many cases of aphasia, there is no clear separation of cortical and subcortical lesions. Two general types of subcortical aphasia are thalamic and those resulting from lesions outside the thalamus. According to Nadeau and Rothi (2001, p. 457):

> In the case of subcortical aphasias stemming from thalamic lesions, the language disorders appear to result from the impact of thalamic dysfunction on cerebral cortical function (i.e., a neural systems disorder). In the case of subcortical aphasias stemming from lesions outside the thalamus, the language disorders reflect either the invisible cortical damage associated with the vascular event that caused the visible subcortical lesion (i.e., a pathological correlate), or they reflect the impact of the subcortical lesion on pathways between the thalamus and language cortex (i.e., a neural systems disorder similar to that in thalamic aphasia).

While subcortical brain structures and neuronal tracts are indirectly involved in language processing, they are not integral to encoding, manipulating, and decoding linguistic codes per se. Consequently, subcortical aphasias are not language disorders in the traditional definition of the term and are primarily auditory perceptual or motor speech impairments.

Progressive aphasia was first identified by Marcel Mesulam in 1982. It is the prolonged, gradual, and subtle language deterioration over at least a two-year period and occurring without signs and symptoms of dementia. Progressive aphasia, also called *primary progressive aphasia*, is not the mental deterioration associated with the decline of language functions such as occurs in Alzheimer's and other insidious diseases affecting cognition. The language deterioration may affect language encoding and motor speech or language decoding resulting in fluent jargon (Kertesz and Munoz, 1997). According to McNeil and Duffy (2001), most patients with progressive aphasia are aware of the language impairments before their family and friends. Davis (2007) notes that progressive aphasia initially impairs a particular language function such as naming, and then it spreads to other language functions.

Atypical aphasias include those resulting from brain tumors, infections, metabolic disorders, head trauma, and damage to the language-dominant right hemisphere in right-handed persons (crossed aphasia). Brain tumors may be benign or malignant and their effects on language functions depend on their size and location in the brain. Until the tumors are removed or reduced in size, the language deterioration can be progressive. However, neurosurgery and other cancer treatments may also damage the brain contributing to the aphasia. Brain infections (viral and bacterial) and metabolic disorders (genetic or acquired) also can cause language deterioration and impairments depending on their neurological effects. Although head traumas may cause the language impairments seen in classic aphasia, frequently they result in atypical aphasic symptoms because of the patient's reduced or impaired consciousness (See Chapter 7). *Crossed aphasia* is the result of brain damage occurring in the right hemisphere of the brain in a person who is definitively right-handed. This rare language disorder occurs in less than 4% of the cases of aphasia and is usually a mirror image of typical left hemisphere profiles (Davis, 2007).

> Crossed aphasia is sometimes referred to as *nondominant aphasia.*

Aphasic Agrammatism

Aphasic agrammatism (AG) is a disorder of grammar. Broadly defined, agrammatism is an impairment, in any modality, of the ability to use and comprehend the rules governing language including phonology and syntax. Patients with aphasic agrammatism have more difficulty with so-called "function" rather than "content" words. Function words, such as articles, pronouns, and conjunctions, serve a grammatical purpose while content words involve lexical or dictionary meanings.

A feature of aphasic agrammatism is *telegraphic speech* where content words are used to the exclusion of function ones. The concept of telegraphic speech is based on the historical practice of telegrams being charged by the word; senders of telegrams would only use the words necessary to carry the basic meaning of the message. An example of telegraphic speech is "I go sleep" for "I want to go to my bedroom and sleep, now." There are two theoretical issues regarding aphasic agrammatism; does it occur because of a central grammatical disorder or because of an overall reduction in vocabulary?

In aphasia, the fundamental language disorder involves encoding and decoding linguistic codes. Consequently, agrammatism includes selective, specific, and isolated grammatical deficits such as impairments using and understanding verbs, prepositions, adjectives, and so forth. However, the "strong version" of this hypothesis is not supported by current research (Berndt, 1998). Because aphasia is also a general reduction of vocabulary, with content words occurring more frequently than function words, disorders of production and comprehension of grammatically correct utterances reflect this overall impoverishment of vocabulary. Aphasic agrammatism, including telegraphic speech, is likely a result of impaired grammatical processing but primarily a consequent of across-the-board vocabulary reduction.

Aphasic Acalculia

Mathematics is considered the universal language. Mathematical symbolic expression, manipulation, and reception involve grammar, syntax, and the symbol-referent relationship of semantics. In addition, when communicating about mathematical functions, conventional words, verbal and graphic, are used to express and understand the information being imparted or received. It is not surprising that the language disorder of aphasia also impairs, more or less, the patient's ability to perform and understand simple and complex mathematics. *Aphasic acalculia* (AC) is the acquired inability to perform or understand mathematical calculations due to brain pathology. *(Dyscalculia* refers to a developmental learning disorder involving mathematical calculations.) Pure or *primary acalculia* occurs in the absence of aphasia and other neurological injury and is less common than aphasic acalculia (Kaplan, Gallagher, and Glosser, 1998). Acalculia is a symptom of the *Gerstmann syndrome* along with agraphia, finger agnosia, and right-left disorientation. However, there is some question whether these four disorders occur in combination with each other in such frequency as to constitute a "syndrome."

Multilingualism and Aphasia

Today, many people are *multilingual*: they speak and understand more than one language. However, there are degrees of multiple language competence and several factors that must be considered in understanding how aphasia affect *polyglots*, people who know and use several languages. According to Pearce (2005), clinical studies show that multiple languages are at least partially represented in different brain areas and aphasia disrupts them differently. Aphasia does not necessarily impair languages with the same degree of severity, and individual patients' recovery patterns vary. Two important factors in addressing multilingualism and aphasia are the age of acquisition and degree of mastery for each language. Language appears to be represented differently in persons who acquire a second language as children compared to those who learn an additional language or languages later in life. Additionally, most polyglots understand later-learned languages better than they can speak them.

Three "rules" of language recovery in polyglot aphasic patients have been proposed: *Pitres, Ribot,* and *Minkowski.* Pitres' rule states that the language most used before the neurological insult will be recovered first and most completely. In Pitres' rule, because of the recent use of one language over another, unparallel recovery will favor the one being used at the time of the brain injury. Pitres' rule could also result from the fact that many patients undergoing treatment do so in the language being used at the time of the neurological injury. Thus, frequent exposure to that language and therapies being conducted in it result in preferential recovery.

Ribot's rule states that the first learned language will be less impaired, recovered first, and relearned most completely. The so-called "mother tongue" will be most resistant to loss and recovered best when compared to secondary languages. The psychological explanation for Ribot's rule is the often stated dictum: "If two memories are of equal strength today, the one first learned will be stronger tomorrow." First learned memories and behaviors are less resistant to loss and extinction.

Minkowski's rule proposes that the language with the strongest affective ties will be least impaired in aphasia and most readily recovered (Paradis, 1998). Minkowski's rule can also include the prestige of the language and its dialectal variations. For example, in Arabic, some dialects are more closely tied to the Koran, giving them more status, and making them resilient to loss and more easily recovered.

Review of the current theories and research on multilingualism and aphasia suggests that there is high variability in preferential loss and recovery patterns of multiple languages. At this time, it is impossible to make universal generalities about how more than one language is represented in the human brain and the effects of aphasia on polyglots.

> "When evaluating the speech and language abilities of clients who speak a dialect of English the clinician should focus on the following: 1) non--dialect-specific aspects of speech and language production; 2) those aspects of communication that are universal such as early developing semantic and pragmatic functions; and 3) dialect-specific forms within linguistic contexts considered to be obligatory in the dialect" (Wyatt, 2002, p. 439).

Aphasic Perseveration and Echolalia

Perseveration is the tendency to continue a mental set or an activity for a longer period of time than is appropriate or warranted by the significance of the stimuli. Perseveration is difficulty shifting from one thought and behavior to another. Although perseveration is not a fundamental problem encoding or decoding linguistic codes, and thus a core aspect of the aphasic syndrome, it is a frequent concomitant symptom. Kaplan, Gallagher, and Glosser (1998, pp. 331-332) address perseveration in the context of attention and executive function: "Perseveration, or the intrusive interference of previous responses, is also a problem for many aphasic patients. Although these processes are not linguistic per se, they may interact with any existing language deficits to undermine the residual adaptive potential." Swindell, Holland, and Reinmuth (1998) report that the tendency to perseverate has not been identified with a specific area of the brain. Benson and Ardila (1998) agree that perseveration can result from damage to many different areas of the brain, however, it is often regarded as a fundamental sign of frontal lobe injury. On a neurochemical level, it is likely that perseveration is caused by a neurotransmitter deficiency, particularly those that inhibit neuronal activity.

In aphasia, there are two types of perseveration: verbal and graphic. Verbal or *recurrent* perseveration is the automatic repeating of the same sound, word, or phrase repeatedly. It is as though the perseverating patient cannot inhibit the same verbal response. Verbal perseveration is apparent during sentence completion drills. When a perseverating aphasic patient is asked to complete the sentence, "The United States of _____," he or she may initially provide the correct response "America." However, because of the inability to shift mentally and behaviorally, the patient may also respond with "America" to the next sentence completion request, "Red, white, and _____." "America" may be offered by the patient for subsequent sentence completions such as "You write with a _____" and "Knife, fork, and _____."

Graphic perseveration is manifest by the patient repeatedly producing the same letter, word, or phrase during writing. The patient may write a legible and correct initial letter of a word, and then his or her writing will trail off to illegible small repeated scribbles or a straight line. The graphic perseveration is the result of the patient being unable to shift mentally and graphically from one task to another.

Echolalia is the unsolicited tendency of the aphasic patient to repeat the last sound, word, or phrase spoken by someone else. Although echolalia is often seen in dementia and traumatic brain injuries, Jon Eisenson (1984) considers it to be a concomitant symptom of aphasia and a manifestation of perseveration. Echolalia may occur when an examiner asks a patient "How are you doing?" In response, the patient may automatically respond with the word "Doing." When asked another question, the patient may again automatically utter the last sound, word, or phrase spoken by the examiner. The patient's thoughts are contaminated by the last utterance spoken by someone else.

The Value and Efficacy of Aphasia Therapy

Four thousand years ago, the ancient Egyptians connected brain injury to impaired communication, and questioned whether neurogenic communication disorders are treatable. Since then, the value of aphasia therapy has oftentimes been a controversial point of contention among neuroscientists, physicians, and therapists. Adding to the controversy, in the 1970s, Medicare included aphasia therapy as a covered rehabilitation service with other third-party providers soon following suit. This resulted in an infusion of millions of dollars into the rehabilitation of aphasic patients. What is most important, in the mid 1900s, the public began to believe that aphasia was therapeutically treatable and demanded that rehabilitation services be available to aphasic patients. Scientifically, the value of aphasia therapy became a heated topic of debate as well-intentioned critics wondered whether language could be restored by therapeutic means, and if so, what groups of aphasic patients benefitted from the therapy. In addition, scientists began to research patterns of recovery, prognostic indicators, and the relative efficacy of specific therapies for particular diagnostic groups of patients.

Historically and today, two scientific issues have prompted debate about the value of aphasia therapy in general and the efficacy of specific treatments to restore language in brain damaged persons. The first issue concerns the irreversibility of brain tissue necrosis. Aphasia is caused by the death of brain tissue due to interrupted blood supply, disease, and injury. Thoughtful people ask the question: "If brain damage is permanent, can aphasic patients be expected to recover lost cognitive functions resulting from it?" The fundamental neurological assumption in the provision of therapies to aphasic patients is that these cognitive, behavioral, and counseling procedures and techniques can reverse the effects of brain tissue death.

The second scientific issue complicating the debate about the value of aphasia therapy concerns *spontaneous recovery*. In aphasia, spontaneous recovery refers to the partial or complete recovery of language without formal or informal medical and rehabilitation intervention. Spontaneous recovery is common in most aphasic patients. Darley (1982, p. 110) notes: "Although severely aphasic patients–those identified as globally aphasic–may constitute an exception, it is commonly expected that aphasic patients will display some remission of their language dysfunction without intervention or formal therapy." Lendrem and Lincoln (1985) found that spontaneous recovery of language abilities in stroke patients continued overtime and the extent of the improvement was not related to age, sex, and aphasia type. With regard to the efficacy of aphasia treatments, the scientific question arises whether the gains seen in language recovery by many aphasic patients are the result of aphasia therapy or simply a result of spontaneous recovery.

Although there are many reasons for spontaneous recovery of language in aphasia, the three primary ones are *diaschisis, collateral circulation,* and *cortical plasticity.* It is likely that all three combine to produce spontaneous return of all or some language in many aphasic patients. Diaschisis is the loss of function in an area of the brain at a distance from the primary site of an acute focal injury but anatomically connected to it. Because of the body's natural tendency to heal itself and a reduction of edema, this disconnect of functional areas is gradually reestablished causing a return of language functions. Collateral circulation creates an alternative route of blood supply. It is the process by which an obstructed artery opens and connects two larger ones or different parts of the same artery. Collateral circulation reroutes blood flow around the blockage to reestablish blood supply to diminished oxygenated areas. Cortical plasticity is the gradual transfer from one location to another of a specific language function. It is a neurological adaptive mechanism to compensate for lost language abilities by adjacent areas assuming alternative functions. There is also the belief that the opposite brain hemisphere assumes lost language-dominant hemisphere functions. To facilitate this hemisphere transfer of language function, some patients are required to write with their non-dominant hands. (Of course, changing handedness may also be required because the dominant hand is no longer functional). The clinical assumption is that writing with the non-dominant hand cause increased neural activity in the non-damaged brain hemisphere.

Today, there are few knowledgeable neuroscientists, physicians, and clinicians who doubt the value of therapy for aphasic patients as a group. Darley (1985, p. 176) reviewed research addressing the efficacy of aphasia therapy using studies with and without treatment control groups, individual cases, additional testimony, and concluded: "Language treatment leads to significant improvement in the majority of cases of aphasia." In addition, he reported that the restoring effect of aphasia therapy is for the most part enduring, and there was generalization to linguistic units and modalities not used as therapeutic stimuli. Aphasia therapy is also valuable psychologically: "The gains that result from treatment are not confined to language functions but are also noted in attitude, morale, appropriateness of affect, and maintenance of social contact" (Darley, 1985, p. 183). In a meta-analysis of 55 studies addressing aphasia treatment, Robey (1998) confirmed that aphasia therapies cause desirable clinical outcomes.

Wineburgh and Small (2004, p. 6) observe in the *ASHA Leader* that while the value of aphasia treatment has been proven, it is still controversial. "In order to explore the future of aphasia treatment, we must first address some significant problems in the current therapeutic approach. Although the efficacy of aphasia treatment has been demonstrated, the very fact that this demonstration continues to be controversial in some quarters shows that the treatment of aphasia, despite its effectiveness, remains unsatisfactory." They state that the reasons for the controversial nature of aphasia therapy are threefold. First, there is poor understanding of the functional changes of the brain during the rehabilitation period. Second, treatment options are limited to external manifestations of the damaged brain structures rather than the structures themselves. Third, goals for patient gains as a result of therapy are too modest meaningfully to affect the patient's quality of life.

To reflect the 21st Century understanding of the evolving nature of aphasia and the importance of ongoing diagnostics, the sections on aphasia evaluation and treatment are combined rather than addressed separately and independently. Below are principles of aphasia evaluation and state-of-the-art treatment based on modern understanding of this neurogenic communication disorder.

> Not all statistically "significant" research results yield clinically "important" information about aphasia.

Principles of Aphasia Evaluation and Treatment

Principle 1: An initial aphasia screening and quick assessment should be conducted rather than a comprehensive diagnostic test.

In the past, before initiating treatment, clinicians conducted one comprehensive aphasia evaluation which included assessment of the modalities affected, description of concomitant symptoms, and analysis of other clinical aspects of the disorder. This evaluation was done early postonset, required several hours of testing, and was often performed over multiple diagnostic sessions. Based on the results of the comprehensive evaluation, the clinician classified the patient's aphasia into one of several diagnostic categories labeling it from a myriad of clinical types. After completion of the testing, treatment objectives and schedules were established based on the results of the comprehensive evaluation and a prognosis provided. Only after this lengthy evaluation did the clinician begin formal treatment basing the therapeutic goals, methods, and procedures on the results of that one initial evaluation. Typically, there were monthly updates of the goals, methods, and procedures, but this initial comprehensive evaluation served as the foundation for the aphasia treatment.

The past widespread clinical practice of conducting one detailed and comprehensive aphasia evaluation before initiating therapy is theoretically and practically unsound, and driven by outdated and unnecessary bureaucratic requirements. The initial formal comprehensive evaluation from which to base treatment becomes more and more clinically irrelevant as time passes because most aphasias evolve over time with significantly changing symptoms. Darley (1982, p. 125) notes: "Longitudinal studies of aphasic patients show that as their modality performances change, so do the gestalts of performance, to which various labels have been applied (Wernicke's, Broca's, conduction, anomic, and so forth)."

Comprehensive testing of patients early postonset is a flawed diagnostic strategy because most patients are not neurologically stable at the time of testing. Medications also affect the patient's presentation of symptoms; some drugs are psychoactivating while others reduce patient responsiveness. Even the time of their administration can cause significant daily fluctuations in symptoms. Because of the fluctuating nature of aphasic symptoms, a brief initial screening test should be administered and therapeutic evaluation should be ongoing and integral to each session. Aphasia therapy is a dynamic process requiring periodic review of objectives, flexible treatment goals, and continuous analysis of therapeutic effectiveness.

The First Bedside Session

Prior to meeting with the aphasic patient, the clinician should briefly review the medical chart to determine the nature of the patient's communication disorder, date of onset, type of neurological injury, and any other pertinent medical information. During the first meeting with the aphasic patient, the clinician greets him or her, establishes rapport, and sets the tone for a productive therapeutic relationship. For the patient, it is encouraging and comforting to know that a health care professional is knowledgeable about aphasia and will provide guidance, support, understanding, and assistance during this difficult time. For the patient with severe aphasia, communicating professional commitment to helping him or her navigate through the complexities of this neurogenic communication disorder is challenging, but necessary none-the-less. It is also desirable to meet with family and friends to discuss their particular concerns and to get additional information about the patient. According to Davis (2007, p. 41), the initial diagnostic questions answered by the clinician during the first visit include: 1) Does the patient have a communicative disorder? 2) If so, is the disorder aphasia? 3) If so, what kind of aphasic disorder does the patient have? 4) Does the patient have other disorders besides aphasia?

Initial Screening and Quick Assessment of Aphasia

Although it is clinically inappropriate to comprehensively assess aphasia early postonset, it is necessary to have an initial general understanding of the patient's language disorder to begin diagnostic therapy. There is no shortage of commercially available screening, bedside, abbreviated, short, and quick aphasia tests. Regardless of whether a formal or informal initial screening and quick assessment is used, it is necessary to obtain and record the patient's relevant medical and background information including occupation, education, family support, and psychological status. The initial screening of aphasia should include a general assessment of the patient's peripheral speech mechanism to determine the presence or absence of apraxia of speech (See Chapter 5) and dysarthria (See Chapter 6).

The patient's basic *language decoding competence* is assessed including the ability to follow verbal multiple step directional commands, point to objects and body parts when named, and answer or indicate "yes" or "no" correctly to questions. *Graphic decoding competence* is assessed for matching printed words with pictures, reading single words aloud, and following written instructions. There should also be a general assessment of the patient's ability to understand and follow gestural commands.

The patient's *language encoding competence* is assessed including his or her ability to describe and name common objects, complete sentences, imitate words and phrases, and express higher level language concepts. The nature of wordfinding and naming disorders are assessed including the types of paraphasias produced by the patient. The patient's fluency and meaningfulness of utterances (jargon) are noted. *Language graphic encoding competence* assessment includes abilities such as writing letters, words, sentences, and to dictation. There should also be a general assessment of the patient's ability to express himself or herself with gestures.

The above screening and quick assessment of the patient's basic communication abilities can be subjectively quantified using a modified Likert scale. On this scale, the patient's abilities are rated on a 1 to 5 continuum. A rating of 1 suggests the patient's abilities are *clearly abnormal or nonfunctional* and 5 indicates *clearly normal or functional.* This scale provides the basis for ongoing diagnostics throughout the course of therapy and is the basis for the Quick Assessment for Aphasia (Tanner and Culbertson, 1999). The above initial screening and quick assessment of the patient's basic communication abilities provides the clinician with adequate information to begin diagnostic therapy.

Principle 2: Every session should include informal and subjective assessments to judge the treatment efficacy.

As reported above, there is continuous evolution of aphasic symptoms in most patients. Other factors are also at work affecting the patient's aphasic symptoms, motivation, and responsiveness to treatment including psychological states such as depression and anxiety (See Principle 4). Additionally, aphasic persons, like all people, have normal fluctuations in their overall interest and energy levels in response to environmental stimulation. There may be hourly, daily, and longer periods of differing levels of interest in the rehabilitation program. This places a premium on ongoing assessment of the patient's motivation and consequent treatment efficacy.

All therapeutic intervention should include ongoing evaluation of the value and efficacy of particular therapeutic procedures and the aphasia therapy program in general. This is not to say that time is set aside in each session to collect data for each goal and objective and analysis of pre and post-therapeutic procedure results. Setting aside valuable clinical time to collect and analyze data does not directly benefit the patient. It is only necessary to assess subjectively and generally the patient's ability to benefit from a particular treatment. This process involves determining a basal and comparing it to post-treatment scores. For example, if a patient is being given a sentence completion exercise, where he or she completes statements such as "Knife, fork, and _____, the clinician should generally and subjectively assess the success rate of the treatment. For example, if 20 such sentence completion exercises are given and the patient responds correctly to 40% of them, the goal during the session is to increase the success rate of the patient's sentence completion abilities. The sets of exercises and drills are evaluated for improvement during the sessions with a goal of achieving a significantly higher success rate.

Principle 3: The patient's ability to *profit from experience* should be assessed for each therapeutic procedure, session, and aphasia therapy in general.

Successful aphasia rehabilitation requires that the patient be on a *level of success*, i.e., he or she succeeds more than fails, and actively achieves meaningful therapeutic gains. Consequently, all aphasia therapeutic intervention is *diagnostic therapy* with a determination of whether the patient meaningfully profits from the aphasia therapy in general and a specific treatment in particular. The ability to profit from experience means that the patient learns from a meaningful therapeutic procedure and can apply that learning to his or her real-life situations. Fundamental to the patient's ability to profit from experience are intact memory capabilities and competent mental executive functions to apply what has been learned outside the context of therapy. Diagnostic therapy should assess whether there has been carryover from session-to-session, day-to-day, and longer periods, and most importantly, generalization to outside situations. If there is insignificant or no improvement over time, the goals and therapeutic procedures should be reevaluated and appropriate adjustment made in the rehabilitation program. If there is consistent failure of the patient to profit from experience, aphasia therapy should be discontinued with reevaluation at a later date.

Principle 4: Every aphasic patient should receive a comprehensive mental health or psychiatric evaluation.

Post-stroke depression in aphasia occurs in as many as 80% of patients (Tanner, 2009; Wineburgh and Small, 2004; Tanner, 2003b; and others). The incidence and prevalence of this major psychological disorder constitutes an integral symptom of the aphasic syndrome.

Clinical depression in aphasia is associated with reduced motivation, lethargy, anxiety, hopelessness, and helplessness. It is psychologically painful for the patient and can lead to suicide. Because of the detrimental effects of depression and other psychological reactions on aphasia rehabilitation, every patient should receive a comprehensive mental health or psychiatric evaluation, and treatment if warranted, including the administration of antidepressants and other psychoactive medications, counseling, psychotherapy, and indirect mental health management as appropriate. Throughout the course of rehabilitation, there should be periodic monitoring of the patient by a mental health care professional familiar with depression and other psychological aspects of aphasia.

Depression in aphasia occurs more often in women than men.

Principle 4: For maximum gains, aphasia therapy should be initiated early, provided intensively, and continue for as long as the patient significantly profits from the services.

Darley (1985), and others, have shown conclusively that for maximum gains, aphasia therapy should be initiated early, provided intensively, and continue for several months. The reasoning behind initiating therapy early is twofold. First, early initiation of aphasia therapy ultimately provides more therapeutic intervention and additional time to achieve goals and objectives. Second, early initiation of aphasia therapy helps reduce the development of negative mental sets and counterproductive behaviors on the part of the patient. Aphasia rehabilitation services should begin as soon as the patient is medically stable with the frequency and length of therapy dependent on his or her ability to profit from experience. According to Cherney and Robey (2001, p. 165), intensive therapy is efficacious and effective: "In an extensive record of clinical findings, aphasiologists have produced many findings in several forms of scientific evidence regarding the questions of treatment efficacy and effectiveness. The body of evidence resulting from each line of research supports the conclusion that treatment of aphasia, particularly intensive treatment, is effective." As long as the aphasic patient is significantly profiting from the services, professional ethics dictate that therapy should continue regardless of funding and payment considerations. However, the frequency of intervention can be reduced to reflect the patient's ability to work independently and with support from family, friends, and other health care professionals.

Principle 5: Aphasia therapy should actively involve the patient's family members, other health care professionals, and the utilization of speech-language pathology assistants.

The question is not "if" aphasic patients' family members should be involved in the treatment program, it is "in what capacity." Typically, family members have frequent daily communicative interactions with aphasic patients, perhaps more than rehabilitation professionals. Knapik (1996, p. 342) addresses the role of the family in the aphasic patient's rehabilitation process and suggests a multidimensional role: "This involves active participation of the family in a process that involves specific assumptions, methods and aims."

Formal and systematic inclusion of the patient's family members in the ongoing evaluation and treatment of aphasia is warranted, necessary, and appropriate for two reasons. First, because the patient's family members likely will frequently communicate with the patient, with proper instruction and direction, their reactions can be productive and result in positive communicative exchanges. This is particularly true for patients discharged to home. Knowledgeable and involved family members can reduce the frustration and verbal impotence associated with this neurogenic communication disorder and facilitate meaningful communication exchanges with the patient. Second, the patient's family members can be valuable sources of continuous and ongoing aphasia therapy; they can be therapeutic extensions of the clinician. Each communication event with the aphasic patient should be considered a therapeutic exchange with family members acting as agents for positive and constructive language change. Baker and Tanner (1990) found a positive correlation between knowledgeable and interactive family members and greater recovery from neurogenic communication disorders at the time of discharge from a regional rehabilitation program.

To provide optimal aphasia therapy, all health care professionals involved with the patient rehabilitation should be knowledgeable about the ongoing evaluation, specific treatment procedures, and they should actively participate in aphasia therapy. Language stimulation and indirect therapies can be provided by physical, occupational, recreational, and other therapists during their respective treatments. For example, while an occupational therapist is working on activities of daily living, language stimulation can be provided by naming clothing, body parts, utensils, food items, actions, and so forth. The goals and nature of these activities can be explained and discussed during rehabilitation team meetings and during therapies. This method of ancillary language stimulation by other rehabilitation professionals is similar to what they provide to traumatic brain injured patients during reality orientation programs and integrated therapy. The utilization of speech-language pathology assistants can also be an efficient and cost-effective method of providing rehabilitation services to aphasic patients. The American Speech-Language-Hearing Association (ASHA, 2006) provides guidelines for the training and utilization of speech-language pathology assistants.

Principle 6: Optimal aphasia treatment procedures are evidence-based.

Ideally, all aphasia therapy would be *evidence-based*. According to the American Speech-Language-Hearing Association (2005) position statement, evidence-based practice is an approach to clinical care and decision-making in which current, *high-quality research evidence* is integrated with practitioner expertise and client preferences. The quality of research can be debated for each study (Ratner, 2006), but generally, high quality research involves the experimental scientific method, replication, and peer-review. The foundation for this method was initially established by John Stuart Mill in his "canons" of induction (Velasquez, 2002). High quality experimental research requires the use of inferential statistics allowing generalizations that go beyond data obtained in the study.

Ideally, evidence-based aphasia treatment practices would be based on the *medical model* for each treatment procedure. In medicine, an applied science that draws from anatomy, physiology, biology, genetics, medicine, and other disciplines, the practitioner prescribes medicines and treatments that have been extensively scientifically tested in several clinical trials. From the scientific evidence, the medical practitioner knows their appropriate application, side effects, and for which type of disorder and patient they are appropriate. To practice rigorous evidence-based aphasia therapy, the clinician would only provide a treatment based on clinical scientific research, preferably with replicated results, showing its efficacy with a particular disorder and patient. There are aphasia therapies meeting the stringent standard of current, high-quality research and providing an evidence-base for their efficacy. They are found primarily in journals and convention presentations and should be used as a treatment of first-choice when available. Unfortunately, there is a dearth of current, high-quality research in aphasia therapy from which to provide an evidence-base for treatment. Of the research available, its inherent heterogeneity is a limiting factor: "The heterogeneity within the pool of studies reporting clinical outcomes limits reliable and valid combinations of data and provides significant challenges for the future development of aphasia therapy research" (Douglas, Brown, and Barry, 2003, pp. 52-53).

> The foundation to all logic is consistency. If an argument is true and valid, it must always be true and valid.

Principle 7: In the absence of current, high-quality research in aphasia therapy, *clinical syllogisms* can provide a logical method of clinical decision making.

According to the *Code of Ethics* of the American Speech-Language-Hearing Association (2003): "Individuals shall evaluate the effectiveness of services rendered and of products dispensed and shall provide services or dispense products only when benefit can reasonably be expected." The most powerful way of determining whether an aphasia therapy can "reasonably" be expected to benefit the patient is through the above scientific method involving inductive logic. However, given the shortage of high quality research, it would be impossible for a clinician to base all aphasia treatment procedures on them. Historically and today, there is simply not enough high quality applied scientific research available to practitioners. According to Tanner and Gerstenberger (1996, p. 328):

> This unfortunate void of research extends to all aspects of clinician-patient interaction including the utilization of workbooks, apraxia and dysarthria drills, word recall assist strategies, techniques for reducing perseveration and bouts of emotional lability, reading and writing rehabilitation, orientation and stimulation and reinforcement techniques. Much of what a practising clinician must do has not been tested empirically. By necessity, therapy is a combination of borrowed teaching strategies from education, psychology, logical inductive and inductive reasoning, commonsense direction and guidance. The limited body of applied research is certainly not desirable, but the practising clinician must perform; he/she does not have the academic luxury to close the lecture with the statement that "all the data are not in."

Even when there is high quality, scientifically-based experimental research available for a particular procedure, speech-language pathologists are more likely to choose a treatment approach based on previous success with it (Royal-Evans and Marcus, 2004).

Clinical syllogisms can provide a method of deductive logical reasoning to determine whether an aphasia treatment procedure can reasonably, that is logically, benefit a particular patient (Tanner, 2006, Tanner, Sciacca, and Cotton, 2005, Lum, 2002). Clinical syllogisms use deductive logic to determine the truth and validity of clinical assumptions. According to Velasquez (2002) in deductive reasoning, if the conclusions drawn are logically based on true evidence in their support, then they are true or probably true in a valid logical argument. In formal deductive logic, a valid argument is one in which the conclusion logically follows the premise and the conclusion is true if the premises are true. There are three clinical syllogisms applicable to aphasia therapy: *clinical intuition, clinical authority,* and *relative application.*

Clinical Intuition

Intuition is automatic instinctive reasoning. Clinical decisions made on intuition are the least robust method of nonscientific knowledge. Without scientific proof, the clinician may rely on his or her clinical intuition that a particular aphasia treatment procedure is applicable to a specific disorder and patient. The clinical intuition syllogism is as follows:

Premise: Clinical intuition can be applied to aphasia treatment procedures.

Premise: My clinical intuition says this aphasia treatment procedure is indicated and appropriate.

Conclusion: This aphasia treatment procedure is indicated and appropriate for this particular disorder and patient.

According to Lum (2002), intuitions are based on introspections, frequently not communicable, and at least partially suspect.

Clinical Authority

Reliance on clinical authority is based on the professional knowledge and expertise of someone or a professional organization. The robustness of this clinical decision is related to the credibility of the authority. The logic for application by authority is as follows (Lum, 2002, p. 25):

Dr. X (a popular or respected individual) claims procedure X works or Factor Y causes Z.

Popularity and respect are qualities that represent endorsement of this person by the community.

Dr. X is valued in the community and therefore Dr. X's ideas must be valid.

Dr. X's ideas must be credible or right.

Based on the above logic, the clinician selects a particular aphasia treatment procedure based on the credibility of the authority. This is the most likely nonscientific approach used by students in clinical practicum based on the authority of the clinical supervisor.

Relative Application

Relative application is the selection of a particular aphasia treatment procedure because its value has been shown with similar cases. Essential to truth and validity of the argument is the similarity of the application across disorders and patients. The argument for using a non-scientifically tested aphasia treatment procedure is as follows:

Premise: Treatment procedure X works with patients in related disciplines.

Premise: Treatments that work with patients in related disciplines can be applied to similar aphasia patients with similar communication disorders.

Conclusion: This aphasia treatment procedure will work with this particular aphasic patient.

> "When one is helping another, both are strong."
> –German Proverb

The following are analytic questions to consider when evaluating nonscientific aphasia clinical procedures (Tanner, 2006; Tanner, Sciacca, and Cotton, 2005):

1. What evidence exists that the premise is based on fact?
2. Is the structure of the argument valid? Does the conclusion logically follow the premise?
3. Does clinical experience with other aphasic patients support the truthfulness of the premise?
4. Does the premise appear congruent and consistent with the nature of aphasia?
5. Does the structure of the clinical syllogism appear logical?
6. Is there a reasonable cause-effect or correlation hypothesis to the syllogism?
7. Does the premise have empirical evidence to support it? Is it, in itself, a logical statement?

Figure 3.2 shows the principles of optimal aphasia therapy.

An initial aphasia screening and quick assessment should be conducted rather than a comprehensive diagnostic test.
Every session should include informal and subjective assessments to judge the treatment efficacy.
The patient's ability to *profit from experience* should be assessed for each therapeutic procedure, session, and aphasia therapy in general.
Every aphasic patient should receive a comprehensive mental health or psychiatric evaluation.
Aphasia therapy should actively involve the patient's family members, other health care professionals, and the utilization of speech-language pathology assistants.
Optimal aphasia treatment procedures are evidence-based.
In the absence of current, high-quality research in aphasia therapy, *clinical syllogisms* can provide a logical method of clinical decision making.

Figure 3.2: Principles of aphasia therapy

Chapter Summary

Aphasia, the acquired loss of language, can be a devastating disorder for the patient and a complex rehabilitation challenge for the clinician. While there are a multitude of aphasia diagnostic categories, labels, and systems, this neurogenic communication disorder can be classified into language encoding and decoding deficits each affecting verbal, graphic, and gestural modalities. Because aphasia often changes in type and affected modality performance, and to measure the ongoing efficacy of therapeutic procedures, diagnostic therapy is conducted in every session. While optimal aphasia treatment procedures are evidence-based, there is a dearth of applied scientifically-based research from which to select therapies. In the absence of high quality evidence-based research, clinical syllogisms can be used as a logical method of treatment procedure selection.

Study and Discussion Questions

1. Provide your own definitions of language and aphasia.
2. Describe the essential parameters of language necessary to any definition of aphasia.
3. List and describe the language encoding disorders.
4. List and describe the language decoding disorders.
5. Compare and contrast the transcortical aphasias.
6. Where is the assumed site of lesion in conduction aphasia?
7. Define and describe subcortical, progressive, and atypical aphasias.
8. Why are mathematical symbolic expression, manipulation, and reception impaired in aphasia?
9. Compare and contrast Pitres, Ribot, and Minkowski's rules with regard to multilingualism and aphasia.
10. Why is echolalia considered an aspect of perseveration?
11. What is spontaneous recovery and why does it occur in aphasia?
12. List and discuss each principle of aphasia therapy.

References

American Speech-Language-Hearing Association (2003). Code of ethics. Retrieved from the World Wide Web on February 7, 2007: http://www.asha.org/NR/rdonlyres/F51E46C5-3D87-44AF-BFDA-346D32F85C60/0/v1CodeOfEthics.pdf

American Speech-Language-Hearing Association (2005). Evidence-based practice in communication disorders [Position Statement]. Retrieved from the World Wide Web on February 7, 2007: http://www.asha.org/members/deskrefjournal/deskref/default.

American Speech-Language-Hearing Association (2006). Frequently asked questions about speech-language pathology assistants (Updated 7/28/06). Retrieved from the World Wide Web on February 7, 2007: http://www.asha.org/about/membership-certification/faq_slpasst. htm (Author).

Baker, M. and Tanner, D. (1990). Recovery from brain insult: Investigation of patient and family adaptation. A paper presented to the annual convention of the Canadian Association of Speech-Language Pathologists and Audiologists, Vancouver, BC.

Beeson, P.M. and Hillis, A.E. (2001). Comprehension and production of written words. In *Language intervention in aphasia and related neurogenic communication disorders* (4th ed.). R. Chapey (Ed). Philadelphia: Lippincott Williams and Wilkins.

Benson, F. D. and Ardila, A. (1996). *Aphasia: A clinical perspective.* New York: Oxford University Press.

Berndt, R.S. (1998). Sentence processing in aphasia. In *Acquired aphasia* (3rd ed.). M. Sarno M. (Ed). San Diego: Academic Press.

Brownell, R. (2000). *Expressive One-Word Picture Vocabulary Test* (3rd ed). Novato, C.A.: Academic Therapy Publications.

Bruer, J. (1999, September). "In search of brain-based education." *Phi Delta Kappan*, 80, 649-657.

Cappa, S. F., Cavallotti, G., and Vignolo, L. (1981). Phonemic and lexical errors in fluent aphasia: Correlation with lesion site. *Neuropsychologia*, 19, 171-177.

Chaika, E. (1974). A linguist looks at "schizophrenic" language. *Brain and Language,* 257-276.

Chapey, R. and Hallowell, B. (2001). Introduction to language intervention strategies in adult aphasia. In *Language intervention in aphasia and related neurogenic communication disorders* (4th ed.). R. Chapey (Ed). Philadelphia: Lippincott Williams and Wilkins.

Cherney, L.R. and Robey, R.R. (2001). Aphasia treatment: Recovery, prognosis, and clinical effectiveness. In *Language intervention in aphasia and related neurogenic communication disorders* (4th ed.). R. Chapey (Ed). Philadelphia: Lippincott Williams and Wilkins.

Damasio, A. R. (1998). Signs of aphasia. In *Acquired aphasia* (3rd ed.). M. Sarno (Ed). San Diego: Academic Press.

Darley, F.L. (1982). *Aphasia*. Philadelphia: W.B. Saunders.

Davis, G.A. (2007). *Aphasiology: Disorders and clinical practice* (2nd ed.) Boston: Pearson, Allyn and Bacon.

Dirckx, J.H. (2001). *Stedman's concise medical dictionary for the health professions* (4th ed.). Philadelphia: Lippincott Williams and Wilkins.

Douglas, J., Brown, L., and Barry, S. (2003). The evidence base for the treatment of aphasia after stroke. In S. Reilly, J. Douglas, and J. Oates (Eds). *Evidence based practice in speech pathology.* London: Whurr Publishers.

Duffy, R.J., Duffy, J.R., and Pearson, K. (1975). Pantomime recognition in aphasic patients. *Journal of Speech and Hearing Disorders*, 18, 115-132.

Eisenson, J. (1984). *Adult aphasia* (2nd ed.). Englewood Cliffs, N.J.: Prentice-Hall.

Goodglass, H. And Kaplan, E. (1963). Disturbance of gesture and pantomime in aphasia. *Brain*, 86:703-720.

Haynes,W. O. and Pindzola, R. H. (2004). *Diagnosis and evaluation in speech pathology* (6th ed.). Boston: Pearson Allyn & Bacon.

Institute of General Semantics. (2007). About General Semantics. Retrieved from the World Wide Web January 21, 2007: http://time-binding.org/institute.htm (Author)

Kearns, K. P. and Elman, R. J. (2001). Group therapy for aphasia: Theoretical and practical considerations. In *Language intervention in aphasia and related neurogenic communication disorders* (4th ed.). R. Chapey (Ed). Philadelphia: Lippincott Williams and Wilkins.

Kaplan, E., Gallagher, R.E., and Glosser, G. (1998). Aphasia-related disorders. In *Acquired aphasia* (3rd ed.). M. Sarno (Ed). San Diego: Academic Press.

Kertesz, A. and Munoz, D.G. (1997). Primary progressive aphasia. *Clinical Neuroscience*, 4, 95-102.

Knapik, H. (1996). Aphasiology and family therapy–development of the subjects. In *Forums in clinical aphasiology*. C. Code and D. J. Müller (Eds). London: UK.

Laakso, M. (2003). Collaborative construction of repair in aphasic conversation. In Goodwin, C. (Ed). *Conversation and brain damage*. Oxford: Oxford University Press.

Lendrem, W. and Lincoln, N.B. (1985). Spontaneous recovery of language in patients with aphasia between 4 and 34 weeks after stroke. *Journal of Neurology, Neurosurgery, and Psychiatry,* Vol 48, 743-748.

Lum, C. (2002). *Scientific thinking in speech and language therapy.* Mahwah, N.J.: Lawrence Erlbaum Associates.

McNeil, M.M. and Duffy, J.R. (2001). Primary progressive aphasia. In *Language intervention in aphasia and related neurogenic communication disorders* (4th ed.). R. Chapey (Ed). Philadelphia: Lippincott Williams and Wilkins.

Marshall, J.C. and Newcombe, F. (1966) Syntactic and semantic errors in paralexia. *Neuropsychologia,* 4, 169-176.

Marshall, J.C. and Newcombe, F. (1973) Patterns of paralexia: A psycholinguistic approach. *Journal of Psycholinguistic Research,* 2, 175-199.

Marshall, R. (1976). Word retrieval behavior of aphasic adults. *Journal of Speech and Hearing Disorders,* 41: 444-451.

Mesulam, M. (1982). Primary progressive aphasia: Differentiation from Alzheimer's disease. *Annals of Neurology* 22: 533-534.

Nadeau, S.E. and Rothi, L.J. (2001). Rehabilitation of subcortical aphasia. In *Language intervention in aphasia and related neurogenic communication disorders* (4th ed.). R. Chapey (Ed). Philadelphia: Lippincott Williams and Wilkins.

Nicolosi, L., Harryman, E. and Kresheck, J. (2004). *Terminology of communication disorders: Speech-language-hearing* (5th ed.). Philadelphia: Lippincott Williams & Wilkins.

Oxford Concise Dictionary (2004). Oxford: Oxford University Press.

Paradis, M. (1998). Acquired aphasia in bilingual speakers. In *Acquired aphasia* (3rd ed.). M. Sarno (Ed). San Diego: Academic Press.

Pearce, J.M.S. (2005). A note on aphasia in bilingual patients: Pitres' and Ribots' laws. *European Neurology*, Vol. 54, No. 3: 127-131.

Ratner, N.B. (2006). Evidence-based practice: An examination of its ramifications for the practice of speech-language pathology. *Language, Speech, and Hearing Services in the Schools*, Vol. 37: 257-267.

Robey, R. R. (1998, February). A meta-analysis of clinical outcomes in the treatment of aphasia. *Journal of Speech, Language, and Hearing Research*, Vol. 41, 172-187.

Roeltgen, D. P. (1993). Agraphia. In *Clinical neuropsychology*, K. Heilman and E. Valencia (Eds). New York: Oxford University Press.

Rosati, G. and DeBastiani, P. (1976). Pure agraphia: A discrete form of aphasia. *Journal of Neurology, Neurosurgery and Psychiatry,* 42: 266-269.

Royal-Evans, C., and Marcus, R. (2004, May). A survey of the use of evidence-based practice in treatment of aphasia. In the 34th *Proceedings of Clinical Aphasiology Conference*, Park City, Utah.

Sarno, J. E. and Gainotti, G. (1998). The psychological and social sequelae of aphasia. In *Acquired aphasia* (3rd ed.). M. Sarno (Ed). San Diego: Academic Press.

Shaywitz, S. and Shaywitz, B. (2007, September). The neurobiology of reading and dyslexia. *ASHA Leader*, Vol. 12, No. 12: 20-21.

Sternberg, R. and Ben-Zeev, T. (2001). *Complex cognition: The psychology of human thought.* New York: Oxford University Press.

Swindell, C., Holland, A. and Reinmuth, O. (1998). Aphasia and related adult disorders. In G. Shames, E. Wiig, and W. Secord (Eds). *Human communication disorders.* Boston: Allyn and Bacon.

Tanner, D. (2001, April). Hooray for Hollywood: Communication disorders and the motion picture industry. *ASHA Leader,* 6(6).

Tanner, D. (2003a) *Exploring communication disorders: A 21ˢᵗ century introduction through literature and media.* Boston: Pearson Allyn & Bacon.

Tanner, D. (2003b, Winter). Eclectic perspectives on the psychology of aphasia. *J. Allied Health: 32:256-260.*

Tanner, D. (2006). *An advanced course in communication sciences and disorders.* San Diego: Plural.

Tanner, D. (2007a). *The medical-legal and forensic aspects of communication disorders, voice prints, and speaker profiling.* Tucson: Lawyers and Judges Publishing.

Tanner, D. (2007b). Redefining Wernicke's area: Receptive language and discourse semantics. *J Allied Health, 36:63-66.*

Tanner, D. (2009). *The psychology of neurogenic communication disorders: A primer for health care professionals.* New York: iUniverse.

Tanner, D. and Culbertson, W. (1999). *Quick assessment for aphasia.* Oceanside, CA.: Academic Communication Associates.

Tanner, D., Culbertson, B, and Secord, W. (2001). *Cheers and jeers: Hollywood and the motion picture industry.* An extended seminar presented to the annual convention of the American Speech-Language-Hearing Association, New Orleans.

Tanner, D. and Cotton, S. (2005). The psychology of global aphasia. (Workshop). *4ᵗʰ Annual Hawaii International Conference on Social Sciences,* Honolulu, Hawaii.

Tanner, D., Sciacca, J. and Cotton, S. (2005). Science and logic in diagnosis and treatment of communication disorders. *4ᵗʰ Annual Hawaii International Conference on Social Sciences,* Honolulu, Hawaii.

Varney, N.R. (1978). Linguistic correlates of pantomime recognition in aphasic patients. *Journal of Neurology, Neurosurgery and Psychiatry,* 41, 564-568.

Velasquez, M. (2002). *Philosophy* (8ᵗʰ ed.). Belmont, CA.: Wadsworth/ Thomson Learning.

Vygotsky, L. (1962). *Thought and language.* New York: MIT Press and John Wiley & Sons.

Webster's New World College Dictionary (4ᵗʰ ed.). Foster City, CA.: Books Worldwide, Inc.

Weinstein, E., Lyerly, O., Cole, M., and Ozer, M. (1966). Meaning in jargon aphasia. *Cortex,* 2: 165-187.

Weinstein, E. and Puig-Antich, J. (1974). Jargon and its analogues. *Cortex,* 10:75-83.

Wertz, R.T. (2000). Aphasia therapy: A clinical framework. In I. Papathanasiou (Ed), *Acquired neurogenic communication disorders: A clinical perspective.* London: Whurr Publishers.

Wineburgh, L.F. and Small, S.L. (2004, April 27). Aphasia treatment at the crossroads: A biological perspective. *The ASHA Leader,* pp. 6-7, 18.

Wood, K. (1971). Terminology and nomenclature. In L. E. Travis (Ed), *Handbook for Speech Pathology and Audiology*. Englewood Cliffs, N.J.: Prentice-Hall.

Wyatt, T.A. (2002). Assessing communicative abilities of clients from diverse cultural and language backgrounds. In D. E. Battle (Ed), *Communication disorders in multicultural populations* (3rd ed.). Boston: Butterworth-Heinemann.

Zimmerman, I., Steiner, V., and Pond, R. (1992). *Preschool language scale-3*. San Antonio, Tx: The Psychological Corporation.

Chapter 4: Neurogenic Perceptual Disorders

> "Language is not simply a reporting
> device for experience but a
> defining framework for it."
>
> Benjamin Lee Whorf

Chapter Preview: This chapter examines the nature of perception and its disorders. There is justification for having neurogenic perceptual disorders as a separate academic and clinical designation of communication disorders. The Sapir-Whorfian hypothesis and its implications for the perception of abstract language are reviewed. In this chapter, audition and auditory-acoustic agnosia are reviewed as they pertain to auditory comprehension. There is also an examination of the types of paraphasia exhibited by the fluent jargon aphasic patient suggesting the level of information input processing involvement. Visual perception, object agnosia, and agnostic alexia are also discussed. In this chapter, principles of treatment for neurogenic perceptual disorder are reviewed.

Perception and Agnosia

Perception is the process of attending to the significance and the routing of salient sensory information for higher cortical processing. Mentally, perception lies between the sensory and associative cognitive functions. Sigmund Freud first coined the term *agnosia* in the late 1800s as a perceptual disorder. Henry Head (1926) recognized the importance of the ability to appreciate the significance of auditory and visual stimuli in the evaluation of aphasia. Benson and Ardila (1998) describe agnosia as a percept without its meaning and a general lack of recognition. Jon Eisenson (1984, p. 10) considers agnosia a frequently occurring disturbance in aphasia: "Such impairments of perception have serious implications for language if they involve auditory or visual modalities or, in the case of blind persons, the tactile modality." While aphasic disorders, to varying degrees, cross all modalities of communication, agnosias are usually limited to one modality.

Narrow definitions of agnosia, based on even narrower definitions of perception, simply define it as a rare disorder of recognition resulting in a patient's inability to identify objects, sounds, or people without sensory transmission deficits usually associated with damage to the parietal lobes. However, broadly and appropriately defined, agnosia is the primary neurogenic perceptual disorder resulting in the patient's inability to attend and appreciate the significance of environmental stimuli in the absence of sensory input deficits. As such, agnosia has across-the-board implications in the diagnosis and treatment of neurogenic communication disorders because perception is fundamental to communication, language, consciousness, and thought.

Perception is a process of selecting, organizing, and interpreting sensory stimulation into a meaningful picture of the world (Nicolosi, Harryman, and Kresheck, 1996).

The Scientific and Clinical Distinction of
Neurogenic Perceptual Disorders

The question may be asked: "Why independently study neurogenic perceptual disorders?" The simple answer to this question is that neurogenic perceptual disorders are a distinct and frequently occurring category of acquired communication disorders requiring differentiated therapeutic objectives and treatment procedures. The scientific and clinical distinction of neurogenic perceptual disorders is a natural evolution in the understanding, diagnosis, and treatment of neurogenic communication disorders.

The history of neurogenic communication disorders is one of diagnostic and treatment refinement. As reported in Chapter 2, the ancient Egyptians, Greeks, and Romans only generally addressed neurogenic communication disorders as a single brain dysfunction resulting from multiple etiologies. Over the following centuries, philosophers, scientists, and clinicians refined the understanding of neurogenic communication disorders by recognizing the importance of different etiologies in their symptomatology. For example, the manifestations of neurogenic communication disorders in traumatically brain injured persons (See Chapter 7) is often, but not always, substantially different from what is seen in patients with single infarct strokes. The same is true for neurogenic communication disorders arising from metabolic disorders, cancer, and other diseases.

> The Edwin Smith papyrus is the first written medical document in history. It is believed to have been written somewhere between 3000-2500 B.C.

Moreover, since the ancient Egyptians, Greeks, and Romans, separating neurogenic communication disorders into distinct categories has gradually become a common academic and clinical pattern. Beginning in the late 1800s and continuing today, motor speech disorders have evolved to a distinct, albeit often co-occurring, manifestation of neurogenic communication disorders, and separate from the impaired language of aphasia. More recently, the category of motor speech disorders has further been differentiated to be inclusive of apraxia of speech and several types of dysarthria. Academically, this refinement of diagnostic and treatment classifications has resulted in university training programs offering separate courses in aphasia, motor speech disorders, and communication disorders resulting from traumatic brain injuries.

Clinically, the proper diagnosis and treatment of neurogenic communication disorders involve separation of language impairments from apraxia of speech, and the differentiation of spastic, flaccid, ataxic, hypokinetic, two types of hyperkinetic, and mixed and multiple dysarthrias. While there is clinical overlap in all neurogenic communication disorders, this conceptual separation more precisely reflects clinical reality. This increased precision in diagnostic and treatment practice has generally improved the rehabilitation of patients with neurogenic communication disorders.

The independent designation of neurogenic perceptual disorders is a further refinement of diagnostic and treatment practices for patients with neurogenic communication disorders. Neurogenic perceptual disorders are distinct and separate from language and motor speech disorders, and should be treated as such academically and in clinical practice. Neurogenic perceptual disorders are frequently core symptoms of the auditory comprehension and reading disturbances seen in patients with neurogenic communication disorders.

Sensation, Perception, and Association

Perception occurs with each of the five senses: *vision, hearing, touch, taste,* and *smell.* Sensation is the detection of environmental stimuli and involves sense organs such as the eye, skin, and ear. Perception, Latin from *percipere* or "to take in completely" is a higher neurological, mental, and psychological level of information processing than sensation. Perception allows awareness of what is sensed and is the first stage of attaching meaning to environmental stimuli.

The act of perception has major psychological and philosophical implications about how individuals view the world and the workings of the human mind. Humans sense environmental stimuli, and through a complex process of applying previous learning to new sensations, they perceptually decide what is brought to conscious awareness. Once information is conscious, it can be associated with previously stored knowledge about the world. Language in general, and semantics in particular, are the highest levels of information processing and association. Perception is an ongoing gestalt of attending to sensory input, determining its saliency, and gating personally important information for higher cognitive association. Humans not only perceive what is sensed, they decide what will be allowed to be processed consciously. Campbell (1982, p. 212) observes that the act of perception is unique and personal: "The organism is linked to the world directly, and evolution has designed this linkage to be a snug fit, the brain being tuned to acquire accurate knowledge of the particular environment the organism inhabits."

Intuition and Perception

Intuition is integrally tied to perception. Intuition is a conscious or partially conscious understanding of the relationship between two or more aspects of reality. Intuition occurs at the perceptual level where a person automatically intuits the answer to a question or perceives the relationship between variables. Usually, intuition is associated with an emotional response ranging from euphoria to a feeling of impending doom. Intuition is appreciating the significance of incoming sensory information, the mental awareness of a perceptual relationship, and routing sense information for higher mental processing. That which is perceived provides the requisite information for higher level thought. Because of the fundamental relationship between perception and thought, no discussion would be complete without addressing the *Sapir-Whorfian hypothesis*. (See Chapters 2 and 3 for a discussion of the effects of aphasia on cognition).

> According to Hicks and Sales (2006), Edgar Allan Poe's, *The Murders in the Rue Morgue*, exposed the American public to the lore of "profiling intuition."

Sapir-Whorfian Hypothesis

In the mid 1900s, Linguists Edwin Sapir and his student Benjamin Lee Whorf addressed the role of language in the perception of reality and thought processes. They studied several languages and cultures, especially Hopi Native Americans, and proposed that humans can only think about reality that has language associated with it and that a society's culture is structured by its language. These are the philosophies of *linguistic determinism* and *linguistic relativism* respectively. Actually, Sapir and Whorf's works are based on the *epistemological* philosophy of Immanuel Kant and particularly the role semantics plays in perception.

Today, it is generally accepted that strict interpretation of the Sapir-Whorfian hypothesis cannot be supported. The extreme view of the Sapir-Whorfian hypothesis, applied by liberal multiculturalists, is that language affects how people sense reality. The often-given illustration for this extreme view of the Sapir-Whorfian hypothesis involves the number of words for snow and the sensation of its different types, textures, colors, consistencies, and so forth. For example, the extreme view of the Sapir-Whorfian hypothesis is that because native Eskimos have many more words for snow than desert-dwellers, they actually sense the reality of snow differently and with more precision. However, commonsense suggest that all normal humans have basically the same sensory mechanisms and share the same time-space reality. To test the extreme view of the Sapir-Whorfian hypothesis, Sternberg and Ben-Zeev (2001) studied how speakers of different languages sense and label the color spectrum. They found that speakers of different languages label colors quite differently, as expected, but no matter the language spoken, a *systematic pattern* of color sensation exists across languages. This study, and others, suggests that sensations are direct links to the environment and all humans, no matter their cultures and languages, sense reality in basically the same way. However, there is theoretical and scientific support for language affecting the nature of perception.

Sensation, the detection of environmental stimuli, does not involve the attachment of meaning to the input. However, the perception of what is detected has meaning for the perceiver. While there are the same auditory, visual, tactile-kinesthetic-proprioceptive, gustatory, and olfactory sensation capabilities among all normal humans regarding the detection of reality, perception is at least partially learned, and as such, there are individual, cultural, and linguistic relativistic variations. While visual sensation of the physical properties of snow is essentially the same for all persons with normal vision, the perception of its salient features is affected by language and learning. For example, a desert-dwelling non-skier and an expert downhill racer both see snow essentially the same; the visible light spectrum is 400,000 to 800,000 cycles per second (Goss, 1982). Nevertheless, the word "powder" to describe a type of snow has more salience, meaning, and importance to the downhill racer. Past learning and what visually is allowed to reach conscious awareness makes the perception of powdered snow more personally relevant to the competitive skier. Similarly, the professional violinist and a non-musician will "hear" the same musical piece, but the former will auditorially "perceive" it more precisely than the latter.

The relationship between auditory perception and *abstract semantics* is complex. Words with concrete, tangible references such as "chair," "dog," and "run," have clear parameters of meaning. Although there is abstraction in all semantics, words referring to concrete, tangible objects and actions have *visual imagery* (or other sensory representation) for them. For example, one can draw a "chair" with the requisite attributes to depict it. However, when auditorially perceiving more abstract words such as "honesty," "truthfulness," and "friendship," there are no clear visual or other sensory tangible references. Therefore, the perceiver's initial determination of what is salient in the words' meanings is relativistic and their *denotations*, their explicit primary meanings, have no such clear-cut semantic properties. There is even more ambiguity about their *connotations*. Connotations include the lexical meanings and the personal associations of the words. Therefore, the perception of these words is highly dependent on previous learning and what the perceiver considers salient about them (Tanner, 2007).

> George Orwell's book, *1984*, used linguistic determinism and relativism in addressing "Newspeak" and "Oldspeak."

Perceptual Salience and Figure-Ground

When referring to perception, *salience* is how noticeable, conspicuous, important, and prominent are aspects of a sensation. Contrasts in saliency are easier to perceive when the variations in the sensations are great. For example, visually it is easier to perceive the differences between very good and extremely poor carpentry, masonry, and landscaping. Auditorially, the difference between a professional and novice violin solo is easy to perceive. However, as the sensory input becomes more similar in their features, perceiving the salient aspects of them is less precise and more dependent on previous learning. *Prior learning* is the determining factor in distinguishing salient features. Using the above carpentry, masonry, and landscaping examples, when a carpenter, bricklayer, and landscaper drive through a neighborhood, each senses the homes with the same visual acuity. However, they perceive them differently based on previous learning. The carpenter is attuned to the quality of the framing, the brick layer perceives fine distinctions in the masonry, and the landscaper appreciates minor aesthetics in the placement of shrubs. These heightened and refined perceptual distinctions occur because each has learned the intricacies of these occupations. The same is true auditorially for the professional violinist. A lifetime of violin training has refined his or her auditory perceptual abilities far beyond what a novice is capable of perceiving.

Perceptual salience and *figure-ground* are fundamentally related. In perception, the *figure* is that to which attention is directed and the *ground* is background information or noise. Figure-ground perception involves both attending to the salient signal, but also the ability to ignore surrounding background or ambient sensations. An example of visual figure-ground perceptual salience is a detective attending to important features of a crime scene while ignoring irrelevant information. According to Hicks and Sales (2006), modern crime scene investigators are popularly thought to possess a *sixth sense* in perceiving what is important and ignoring or relegating to secondary importance all other information. Connoisseurs perceive learned important aspects of wines related to their taste and bouquet, and can identify vintages based on their salient features. Tactile figure-ground distinctions occur when a person searches for keys in a pocket or a visually-impaired individual attends to the meaning of raised dots while reading Braille. In the auditory mode, figure-ground is illustrated by the *cocktail party phenomenon*.

The cocktail party phenomenon is the perceiver's ability to attend to various conversations during a group event. He or she selectively attends to a particular conversation while ignoring others. The cocktail party phenomenon can occur without the listener moving his or her head and ears, and is purely an auditory perceptual effect. Through a process of selectively determining what is salient, the perceiver can attend to one conversation and partially or completely ignore competing ones. This can be done *serially*; the listener attends to one conversation, and then another, and so on. Also during a group gathering, auditory figure-ground salience is prompted when someone speaks the listener's name and he or she automatically tunes out other conversations to perceive what is being said.

An *optical illusion* is a type of misleading visual-ground perception. An optical illusion is a discrepancy between a physical measurement and a percept.

The Thalamus and Perception

The *thalamus* is called the *gatekeeper* of sensory information; it is a relay station for the visual, auditory, tactile-kinesthetic-proprioceptive, and gustatory sense information. The thalamus is about the size of a golf ball and is found at the rostral end of the brainstem. It is part of the diencephalon, consists of grey matter, and is hemispheric. It directly or indirectly receives sensory impulses, except olfaction, and routes the information to higher mental centers (Zemlin, 1998). Nadeau and Rothi (2001, pp. 457-458) succinctly review its relay function:

> For example, visual information is transmitted from the retinas via a specific thalamic nucleus, the lateral

geniculate body (LGB), to the primary visual cortex (calcarine cortex) in the occipital lobes. Auditory information is relayed through a chain of nuclei within the brainstem to another thalamic nucleus, the medial geniculate body, from whence it is transmitted to the primary auditory cortex (Heschl's gyrus) on the dorsal surface of the temporal lobe deep within the Sylvian or lateral fissure of the brain. Somatosensory information is relayed by two major pathways within the spinal cord and brainstem to two specific thalamic nuclei, ventral posteromedial (subserving the face), and ventral posterolateral (subserving the body), from which it is then relayed to the somatosensory cortex on the surface of the cerebral hemispheres.

According to Chusid (1973) and others, the thalamus is a crucial structure in the perception of some types of sensations. The thalamus and the *cerebral cortex* work in conjunction to decide what is perceived. It is an interactive process where cortically processed and stored information allows the thalamus and other nervous system structures to gate and route sensory stimuli for higher mental processing and conscious awareness of some or all of the sensory information. "The to-and-fro sensory pathways between the thalamus and cerebral cortex are so numerous, and the two structures so interdependent, that it is sometimes difficult to assign a sensory deficit to the thalamus or the sensory cortical areas of the cerebrum" (Love and Webb, 1996, p. 39).

> The thalamus relays sensory information to various special cortical areas. It is an important area for receiving primitive impulses of pain, temperature, and gross touch.

Some scientists and clinicians consider thalamic-based communication disorders to be a category of *subcortical aphasia*. As discussed in Chapter 3, subcortical aphasias are thought to result from damage to the structures below the cerebral cortex especially the thalamus and the adjacent white matter tracts. While some authors label subcortical aphasia as a "language disorder," they do so only in the broadest definition of the term. They include sensation and perception in the definition of language, postulate invisible cortical damage, or broadly consider subcortical aphasia a *neural systems disorder*. Davis (2007, p. 38) observes that subcortical aphasias have more sensory and motor impairments than *classical syndromes*: "In general, there is some disagreement over whether forms of subcortical language disturbances are genuine aphasia syndromes or are merely similar to these syndromes."

Fundamental Auditory Perceptual Requisites

Before discussing auditory neurogenic perceptual disorders, reviewing the five *general auditory perceptual requisites* is necessary. The distinction between sensation and cursory perception is not absolute, however, and the following are the primary requisites for higher level auditory perceptual processing (Tanner, 2007; Tanner, 2006). First, the listener *detects* sound emanating from the speaker. This involves the hearing mechanism transforming sound waves into mechanical energy at the level of the middle ear and to hydraulic energy at the level of the cochlea. The organ of Corti transforms the hydraulic energy into neural impulses via cranial nerve VIII. Second, the listener attends to the *environmental sound* coming from the speaker and ignores competing olfactory, visual, gustatory, and tactile-kinesthetic-proprioceptive sensory information. Third, the environmental sounds are separated into *speech* and *nonspeech categories* for different higher level perceptual processing. Fourth, the listener *selectively attends* to the speech sounds in three-dimensional space, length, breadth, and depth, and also temporal factors of rate and recency of utterances. The final auditory perceptual requisites are *identification* and *gross discrimination* of vowels and consonants for the determination of the language and dialect spoken. These five fundamental perceptual requisites are necessary to attach perceptual meaning to the auditory input and routing it for higher mental and cortical processing. Table 4.1 shows the general auditory perceptual requisites.

Table 4.1: General Auditory Perceptual Requisites

Sound Detection	Sense of Hearing
Selective Attention	Focus on Salient Feature
Separation of Environmental Sounds into Categories	Speech Detection
Sound Localization	Speech Localization in Time and Space
Identification and Gross Discrimination of Speech Sounds	Attempt to Determine Language Spoken; Gross Vowel and Consonant Perception

Neurogenic Auditory Perceptual Disorders

Neurogenic auditory perceptual disorders are not the result of hearing loss or deafness nor are they the *central auditory processing disorders* typically seen in children. Central auditory processing disorders in children is a broad, and often ill-defined, category of communication disorders. They involve impaired recognition and use of language that is not consistent with intelligence or age (Martin, 1997). Children with central auditory processing disorders primarily have impaired attention to auditory stimuli and reading comprehension deficits. "These are disorders that may be more accurately considered language disorders that involve deficits in the perception and processing of phonetic or phonological information" (Schwartz, 2002, p. 170).

Neurogenic auditory perceptual disorders involve disruptions in the process of attending, appreciating the significance, interpreting, and routing salient auditory sensory information for higher mental and cortical processing. *Auditory* and *acoustic agnosias* are the primary disorders of auditory perception seen in neurogenic communication disorders. Agnosia, Greek for "non-knowing" or "not knowing," is a general category of perceptual disorders involving the inability to attend and appreciate the significance of environmental stimuli without sensory input deficits. Technically, auditory agnosia involves defective perception of speech and environmental sounds while acoustic agnosia is limited to defective speech perception. Acoustic agnosia is sometimes erroneously labeled *pure word deafness*; it is rarely "pure" and often seen in aphasia, seldom limited to "words," and never "deafness" in the traditional, clinical definition of the term.

The auditory comprehension disorders in aphasia can be divided into those that are primarily perceptual and those resulting from *semantic association deficits*. This scientific and clinical distinction is necessary because the therapeutic goals and treatment procedures for neurogenic auditory perceptual disorders are fundamentally different from those for non-perceptual symptoms of aphasia. The primary treatment goals and objectives for semantic association deficits involve relearning verbal *symbol-referent semantic relationships* for recognition and recall. The primary treatment goals and objectives for neurogenic auditory perceptual disorders are improving *auditory attention, appreciation of the significance of auditory input, perceptual interpretation*, and the *routing* of salient auditory sensory information for higher mental and cortical processing. Albert, Sparks, von Stockert, and Sax (1972) suggest that there may be two central auditory mechanisms: *linguistic* and *nonlinguistic*. When evaluating and treating the auditory comprehension deficits in neurogenic communication disorders, it is necessary to learn whether the impairments are *predominantly* perceptual, semantically associative, or a result of impairments of both the perception and association. Although these disorders converge and overlap, each will be discussed separately for theoretical and clinical utility.

> *Intermittent Auditory Perceptual Disorders*, a concept advanced by Hildred Schuell, involve random and sporadic auditory processing deficiencies.

Auditory Agnosia and Amusia

Patients with *auditory agnosia* have normal abilities to detect sound; they are not deaf or hard-of-hearing. The receptive disturbance involves all auditory input including speech perception (See below). Patients with auditory agnosia may misperceive environmental sounds such as fire alarms, telephones, birds chirping, and so forth. According to Benson and Ardila (1996), individuals with auditory agnosia can understand spoken language but not recognize environmental sounds. Most of the published research on auditory agnosia involves attempts to localize it to particular areas of the brain with results ranging from damaged subcortical regions to the temporal and parietal lobes of either hemisphere. In a review of 48 studies conducted on auditory and related agnosias from 1972 to the present, more than 95% focused on localization issues. Remarkably, most of the studies localized auditory and related agnosias to different parts of the brain. Poor research design plagues the localization research on auditory agnosia, especially concerning etiology, subject selection, and absent or vague definitions of perception.

Amusia is considered a specific type of auditory agnosia. Winner and Karolyi (1998, p. 375) explain the relationship of language to music: "Music bears many parallels to language. Both involve a written notation and are based on combinatorial rules. In addition, both involve more than one role: speaker, writer, reader, or listener (language), and performer, composer, critic, or listener (music). Each role can be selectively impaired." A patient with amusia has difficulty or the inability to recognize and produce musical tones and rhythms in the absence of hearing loss or deafness. Amusia can occur with or without aphasia and is inclusive of *tone deafness*. Tone deafness is the inability or impaired ability to perceive differences between musical notes and to produce them correctly. Tone deafness can be from a lack of musical training and also neurological injury. Amusia has been linked to damage to the right temporoparietal lobes (McFarland and Fortin, 1982), but it can also occur from damage to subcortical and cortical structures of either brain hemisphere.

Speech Perception

Several theories explain how humans perceive speech: *bottom-up versus top-down, active versus passive, autonomous versus interactive, interactive-activation, event perception, lexical neighborhood activation,* and *motor* (Kent, 1997). All theories of speech perception recognize that the sense of hearing provides the raw energy for speech perception. Consequently, a particular person's hearing acuity affects the process of speech perception and what he or she ultimately perceives. *Data-driven theories* of speech perception, sometimes called the *bottom-up theory* emphasizes the importance of raw acoustic data for speech perception. And as discussed above, all perception, including speech perception, also involves attention to the signal, attachment of meaning to the input, either conscious or subconscious determination of its salience and importance, and routing to higher levels for processing based on previous learning. Therefore, speech perception is both a bottom-up and a top-down process. It is also influenced by learned expressive articulation gestures as postulated by the *motor theory of speech perception.*

The motor theory of speech perception ties expressive articulation gestures of the speaker to the goals of speech perception. Liberman and Mattingly (1985, p.1) summarize the revised theory: "According to the revised theory, phonetic information is perceived in a biological distinct system, a 'module' specialized to detect the intended gestures of the speaker that are the basis for phonetic categories. Built into the structure of this module is the unique but lawful relationship between the gesture and the acoustic patterns in which they are variously overlapped." According to Kent (1997, p. 386), the motor theory of speech perception recognizes that the syllable is the fundamental unit of speech perception and there are five "special" properties:

1. The acoustic signal of speech represents a substantial restructuring of the phonetic message.

2. Information on successive speech sounds is transmitted in parallel, in a kind of shingling of phonetic features. At a given instant, the acoustic signal may carry information on more than one phoneme.

3. The parallel transmission permits speech to be understood at rates of up to 30 phonetic segments per second.

4. The phonetic units do not have a one-to-one correspondence with the acoustic signal of speech.

5. Although the acoustic signal is not invariantly related to the phonetic message, the motor commands that control the articulators are invariant. This is the *sine qua non* of the "motor theory" of speech perception. The essence of this theory is that speech is understood in terms of how it is produced; in other words, articulation is the referent for perception.

Based on current theories of speech perception, the neurogenic perceptual disorder of acoustic agnosia is the disruption of the perceiver's ability to attend to the important, salient elements of the speech acoustic signal, disruption of the ability to attach perceptual meaning to the distinctive phonetic properties of the syllable, and the deficits routing the utterance for association at higher mental and cortical levels. As such, acoustic agnosia may be a fundamental disorder in all neurogenic auditory comprehension disorders.

> According to Kent (1997), the speech signal consists of four basic types of quality information woven together: phonetic, affective, personal, and transmittal.

Levels of Neurological Deficits and Paraphasias

Three types of impaired speech output are generally recognized in patients suffering from aphasic verbal decoding disorders with fluent jargon: 1) literal phonemic approximation paraphasia–the alternate word phonemically resembles the desired one; 2) verbal semantic association paraphasia–a semantic relationship; and 3) random neologistic paraphasia–no apparent phonemic or semantic relationship between the alternative and desired word. Odell, McNeil, Rosenbek, and Hunter (1991) found that fluent conduction aphasic subjects displayed a different vowel error pattern, i.e., more substitutions than distortions, more errors in polysyllabic than monosyllabic words, and more errors in the initial positions of words compared with subjects with motor speech disorders (apraxia of speech and ataxic dysarthric speakers). This study, and the others discussed above addressing site of lesion in verbal-acoustic agnosia, suggest that the output of the fluent jargon aphasic patient is indicative of the level of verbal input processing impairments (See Table 4.2). The types of paraphasias exhibited by the fluent jargon aphasic patient reflect the level of involvement: perceptual, verbal association, or global cognitive (dynamic). Of course, many patients suffering from aphasic verbal decoding disorders and fluent jargon output have multiple types of paraphasias suggesting more than one level of disruption especially in traumatic brain injuries and large or multiple infarcts.

Table 4.2: Levels of Neurological Deficits

Input	Output
Speech Perception	Literal Phonemic Approximation Paraphasias
Verbal Association	Verbal Semantic Association Paraphasias
Dynamic Inner Speech	Random Neologistic Paraphasias

Patients who produce literal phonemic approximation paraphasias, i.e., phonemically similar but erroneous words for the desired ones such as "fell" for "smell," "fun" for "run," or "kun" for "gun," have speech perception deficits. As noted in the motor speech theory of speech perception, speech is understood in terms of how it is produced and articulation is the referent for perception. Therefore, the neurological deficit is at the perceptual level where the patient perceives speech as being produced with literal phonemic approximations and consequently his or her articulation reflects this impairment. Patients with verbal semantic association paraphasias produce semantically related words for the appropriate ones such as "car" for "truck," "hand" for "foot," or "chair" for "table." These inaccurate circumlocutions represent verbal association deficits where the patient is attempting to select from his or her disordered lexicon the appropriate word for expression. Patients who produce random neologistic paraphasias, where there is no apparent phonemic or semantic relationship between the substituted and appropriate words, have high level cognitive defects affecting the fabric of language. Patients who produce neither verbal semantic association nor literal phonemic approximation paraphasias engage in random neologistic paraphasias and have high level cognitive impairments affecting verbal-cognitive processing (inner speech) and dynamic aphasia (Luria, 1974, 1970, 1966, 1964, 1958). In effect, these patients have lost structured verbal associations and their random neologistic paraphasia reflects this widespread cognitive deficit. Disorders of speech perception can occur at the attentional level where the patient has difficulty focusing on the auditory stimuli and/or result from deficits attaching meaning to the input and routing it for higher levels for processing.

Fundamental Visual Perceptual Requisites

Visual perceptual disorders are not the result of vision acuity deficits or blindness. However, the sense of vision provides the raw energy for visual perception and more than one-third of elderly patients have some visual acuity deficits (Atkins, 1998). Objects in the environment reflect light to the eyes which is detected by the rods and cones of the retina. The detection of light is dynamic, and according to Campbell (1982), it is never static from one moment to the next; light dims or brightens and the observer moves from one position to the next. From the retina, the neural energy is transmitted along the *optic nerve*, cranial nerve II, to the thalamus and higher brain centers. According to Love and Webb (1996, p. 96) "The fibers from the retina of each eye originate from two different areas on each retina. The retinal fibers can be thought of exiting either as temporal fibers–that is, as coming from the lateral half of the retina nearest the temple–or as nasal fibers, which originate from the lateral half nearest the nose." At the optic chiasm, the nasal fibers from each eye decussate while the temporal fibers do not decussate. In communication, the sense of vision is involved in comprehending facial expressions, body gestures, and reading. Visual perception lies between the sense of vision and higher level visual association processes.

> The vestibular mechanism is closely tied to extrinsic eye muscles. Coordination between extrinsic eye muscle movements and the vestibular mechanism preserves stability of visual perception as a person moves about.

Neurogenic Visual Perceptual Disorders

Several types of visual agnosia have been identified including prosopagnosia (faces), color (colors and hues), drawing (objects, complex scenes, and schematics), simultanagnosia (multiple scenes), and visual-spatial (topographical concepts). There are two primary visual perceptual disorders in neurogenic communication disorders: *visual object agnosia* and *agnostic alexia*. When visual perceptual disorders occur with aphasia, they likely are not specific to one type of agnosia although they are usually modality-specific. "Visual agnosias may be specific for objects, representations, geometric forms, colors, letters, words, or other specific configurations. It is unlikely, however, that an individual will have an agnosia for pictures and not for objects, for letters and not for words, or for single words and not for words in context" (Eisenson, 1984, p. 12).

Lissauer (1890) first classified visual agnosias as *apperceptive* or *associative*. Apperceptive visual agnosia fits the definition of a perceptual disorder involving the modality-specific inability or impaired ability to attend, appreciate, interpret, and route salient sensory information for higher mental and cortical processing. Associative visual agnosia is a higher level language-based disorder primarily involving anomia and verbal recall. To add to the chaos of classification in neurogenic communication disorders, some authorities recognize *optic aphasia*. "Some patients experience naming failure restricted to the visual modality (modality-specific), as in visual agnosia. However, they may be able to describe the function of viewed objects, sort objects into categories, or gesture the appropriate use for the object they are unable to name, arguing against a visual agnosia in which meaning is not appreciated for viewed objects" (Raymer and Rothi, 2001, p. 524). In the modern definition of perception and language, associative visual agnosia and optic aphasia are language-based disorders involving visual input and impaired verbal expression, and they are not perceptually-based disorders.

Visual Object Agnosia

Visual object agnosia is the inability or impaired ability to perceive the salience, importance, and function of an object in the absence of visual acuity deficits. Cambier, Signoret, and Bolgert (1989) broadly define three visual object agnosias: *aperceptive, associative,* and *asemantic.* In aperceptive visual object agnosia, the patient's visual perception is poor and with morphological errors; the disorder concerns visual information processing that is necessary for identifying the formal representation of the object. While it is acknowledged that the boundaries of perception and association overlap, aperceptive visual object agnosia fits the definition of a perceptual disorder and the associative and asemantic categories are primarily language-based disturbances. So-called associative and asemantic visual object agnosias involve naming, verbal recall, and the visual-verbal symbol-referent relationship, and as such, are aphasic language disorders and not primarily perceptual in nature.

In visual object agnosia, the patient's "morphological" disorder concerns the perception of the object in three-dimensional space giving cues to its salience, importance, and function. The deficits involve perception of an object's lines and contours, surface and depth contrasts, and cues to its movement and functional capabilities. From the salient visual sensory information, the perceiver attaches meaning to the visual input, appreciates the significance of it, interprets its fundamental morphology, and routes important information for higher mental and cortical processing. In patients with neurological disorders, an example of visual object agnosia is the placing of a spoon or other eating utensil in a glass of water, and the patient sucking from it as if it were a straw. Obviously, the patient does not visually appreciate the significance of the eating utensil. This act may show a perceptual disturbance, aperception, or a higher level cognitive deficit involving associative functions (associative agnosia). If the patient cannot name the object or has problems recognizing the name, he or she suffers from semantic impairments (asemantic agnosia). Of course, patients who do not appreciate the significance of eating utensils may misperceive, inappropriately associate, and also may be semantically impaired.

> Recognition of a visual stimulus is accomplished by comparing it with other items in visual memory.

Agnostic Alexia

In Chapter 3, the graphic decoding disorder, aphasic alexia, was addressed. In aphasic alexia, a language disorder, the reading impairments involve semantic association errors, e.g., deep or central alexia. Agnostic alexia, sometimes called surface alexia, is a visual perceptual disorder where the patient has difficulty spelling and "sounding out" letters and converting them to words. Agnostic alexia is a perceptual impairment involving attention, interpretation, and routing of salient grapheme information for letter-to-sound conversion, i.e., grapheme to phoneme transition. According to Patterson and Behrmann (1997), some patients display marked discrepancies in perceiving letters and converting them to speech sounds for typical spelling-sound correspondences (e.g., toad, mint, profile) versus atypical spelling-sound correspondences (e.g., pint, broad, island). As expected, most alexic patients have more difficulty reading atypically spelled words than those with typical pronunciation. Both surface and deep alexia may co-occur and also be complicated by the visual acuity disorder *homonymous hemianopsia* and *visual neglect* (See Chapter 3).

The graphic processing disorder in agnostic alexia involves the inability to recognize letters visually and access their phoneme auditory memory engrams. Letters, whether handwritten, typed, or seen on a wordprocessor are misperceived. Their salient sizes, shapes, forms, and contours are not perceived as important and consequently meaning is not attached to them. To the patient, the letter symbols, graphemes, have no more meaning than random line scribbles, drawings, shapes, and forms. Consequently, the patient with agnostic alexia, in the absence of visual acuity deficits, does not attach meaning to the graphemes and consequently is unable to retrieve the stored memory of the phonemes for sounding out and spelling-to-sound conversions. The visual perceptual disruption may occur at the attention, interpretation, and routing of salient grapheme information levels of visual perception. Of course, with many neurogenic patients with reading disorders, even when letters are perceived correctly, the words may not be associated meaningfully; they have lost the visual symbol-referent relationship. There is no clear-cut boundary between visual perception and association for reading purposes.

> The trigeminal cranial nerve conveys motor impulses downward and touch impulses upward.

Tactile Agnosia

Tactile agnosia, also called *astereognosis*, is a perceptual disorder related to the sense of touch. It is primarily relevant to patients with neurogenic communication disorders who are visually impaired and rely on the sense of touch for reading Braille. Because of the reliance on touch by these patients, tactile agnosia reduces or eliminates the ability to read. In other patients, tactile agnosia may impair the ability to recognize keys, coins, and other objects in a pocket or purse purely by the sense of touch. *Finger agnosia* is an impairment in the ability to name and differentiate among the fingers of either hand of the self or others (Gerstmann, 1940). It may be a symptom of the *Gerstmann syndrome* along with agraphia, acalculia, and right-left disorientation. However, as discussed in Chapter 3, the Gerstmann syndrome may not be a clinical entity and constitute a syndrome.

Principles of Neurogenic Perceptual Disorders Evaluation and Treatment

Principle 1: Neurogenic perceptual disorders are a distinct designation of communication disorders and as such require separate treatment objectives and procedures.

Neurogenic perceptual disorders, while often co-occurring with aphasia, apraxia of speech, and the dysarthrias, are neither language nor motor speech impairments. As discussed in Chapter 3, the language disorder of aphasia requires identifying the disordered language competence and performance parameters in each modality. The goal is to relearn and deblock expressive and receptive language. The primary treatment objective in apraxia of speech is to relearn voluntary control of the motor speech mechanism, particularly articulation. It is necessary to evaluate dysarthria to determine the type of paralysis, i.e., flaccid and spastic dysarthria, and to structure treatments to minimize their effects on speech production. Concerning the dysarthric movement disorders, i.e., ataxic, hypokinetic, and hyperkinetic dysarthrias, the treatment objectives are to improve speech coordination, prosody, and to decrease or eliminate unwanted movements during speech production. Motor speech disorders and their treatment principles are discussed in Chapters 5 and 6. The treatment of neurogenic perceptual disorders involves maximizing attention to visual and auditory sensory stimuli and relearning salient features for routing to conscious attention.

Principle 2: Treatment objectives for neurogenic communication disorders include addressing visual and/or auditory acuity requisites.

Fundamental to visual and auditory perception is the patient's ability to attend to incoming stimuli. The patient's visual and auditory sensory systems must have the acuity to permit undistorted information available for perception. Salience training involves improving selective attention to reduce figure-ground disorders and to learn to focus on important auditory and visual features of the stimuli which are based on sensory acuity. The patient is taught to separate environmental sounds and visual imagery into linguistic and nonlinguistic categories requiring optimal visual and/or auditory acuity. Hearing aids, cochlear implants, glasses, surgeries, medications, and other treatments should be made available to patients with neurogenic perceptual disorders to minimize sensory impairments.

Principle 3: While perceptual disorders do not influence reality detection, they do affect cognitive representation and processing.

Hillis (2001) proposes a cognitive neuropsychological approach to the treatment of neurogenic communication disorders. There are two basic assumptions to this approach making it applicable to the evaluation and treatment of neurogenic perceptual disorders.

> First, the universality assumption states that everyone has essentially "the same" cognitive processes. Certainly, there may be different modes of learning and thinking that reflect variable reliance on one type of processing relative to another, but we all start out with the same types of mental representations and processes. Second, the "transparency assumption" states that brain-damaged patients also have basically the same cognitive processes, except for a focal modification at some level(s) of representation or processing, "transparently" revealed by the pattern of performance in various tasks (Hillis, 2001, p. 515).

Brain damage does not result in fundamentally new types of mental representations or operations. Consequently, in neurogenic perceptual disorders, treatment objectives and procedures can be based on established learning theories for developing auditory and visual perception in normal persons.

Principle 4: Treatment procedures for neurogenic perceptual disorders include auditory and visual figure-ground therapies.

Integral to perception are the patient's ability to localize and selectively attend to visual, speech, and general auditory stimuli. This ability to separate the "figure," that which is personally important to the perceiver, from the "ground," ambient and personally insignificant information is a primary therapeutic goal in the treatment of neurogenic perceptual disorders. Included in this aspect of treatment are the development of sound and visual stimuli localization and the improvement of selective attention based on the patient's perceptual deficits.

Principle 5: The treatment of auditory agnosia involves attending to nonspeech auditory signals and salience training.

Auditory agnosia is more likely to occur in patients with neurogenic communication disorders arising from traumatic brain injury, dementia, and multiple infarct strokes particularly those who have clouding of consciousness and stupor. The treatment of auditory agnosia includes training the patient to detect and localize nonspeech environmental sounds. Detection training involves increasingly directing the patient's attention to important auditory stimuli. Localizing sound includes selectively attending to the direction sound is emanating, temporal factors such as recency, and to categorize auditory stimuli, e.g., speech, nonspeech, television, etc.

> Salience: Qualities of a stimulus that stand out relative to neighboring items.

Principle 6: The treatment of acoustic agnosia involves attending to speech signals and salience training.

Patients with co-occurring auditory agnosia require therapies to direct attention to important auditory stimuli, sound localization, and categorization of nonspeech and speech stimuli. Therapies for patients with acoustic agnosia include attending to salient phonetic categories of the speech acoustic signal and attachment of meaning to distinctive phonetic properties of the syllable. Essentially, the patient with acoustic agnosia is taught to perceive salient phonetic aspects of speech stimuli and to attach auditory meaning to them.

Principle 7: The treatment of visual object agnosia involves attending to the physical parameters of objects and salience training.

Therapies for visual object agnosia involve addressing the morphological aspects of objects in three-dimensional space. The patient is taught to attend to salient physical cues about important environmental objects including their lines and contours, surface and depth contrasts, movement, and functional capabilities.

Principle 8: The treatment of agnostic alexia involves attending to letters and other graphemes and salience training for reading purposes.

Therapeutic goals in the treatment of agnostic alexia are to train the patient to spell, sound out letters, and convert the auditory information to words. The primary goal is to attach meaning to graphemes and retrieve stored memory of the phonemes, or in the absence of stored meanings, to create new ones. Objectives include attention to salient graphemes and the interpretation of them for routing to conscious awareness during reading. Stimuli include handwritten and typed graphemes, and words on computer screens. Figure 4.1 shows the principles of optimal neurogenic perceptual disorders therapy.

Neurogenic perceptual disorders are a distinct designation of communication disorders and as such require separate treatment objectives and procedures.
Treatment objectives for neurogenic communication disorders include addressing visual and/or auditory acuity requisites.
While perceptual disorders do not influence reality detection, they do affect cognitive representation and processing.
Treatment procedures for neurogenic perceptual disorders include auditory and visual figure-ground therapies.
The treatment of auditory agnosia involves attending to nonspeech auditory signals and salience training.
The treatment of acoustic agnosia involves attending to speech signals and salience training.
The treatment of visual object agnosia involves attending to the physical parameters of objects and salience training.
The treatment of agnostic alexia involves attending to letters and other graphemes and salience training for reading purposes.

Figure 4.1: Principles of neurogenic perceptual disorders therapy

Chapter Summary

Neurogenic perceptual disorders are a distinct category of neurogenic communication disorders. The primary disorders of perception are visual, auditory, and acoustic agnosias although individuals who read Braille may be negatively affected by tactile agnosia. Because these perceptual disorders are often co-occurring in neurological injury, they are treated separately with goals reflecting their perceptual nature. There are eight principles of treatment of neurogenic perceptual disorders addressing localizing visual and auditory stimuli, figure-ground discrimination training, and perceptual salience.

Study and Discussion Questions

1. Define perception and agnosia.
2. Should neurogenic perceptual disorders be a separate clinical distinction in the general category of neurogenic communication disorders? Explain and defend your answers.
3. Describe sensation, perception, and association.
4. Describe the Sapir-Whorfian Hypothesis.
5. Describe perceptual salience and figure-ground.
6. Describe the function of the thalamus in perception.
7. List and discuss the fundamental auditory perceptual requisites.
8. Describe the auditory perceptual disorders.
9. Explain the motor theory of speech perception.
10. List and discuss the neurogenic visual perceptual disorders.
11. List and discuss the principles of treatment for neurogenic perceptual disorders.

References

Albert, M.L., Sparks, R., von Stockert, T., and Sax, D. (1972). A case study of auditory agnosia: Linguist and non-linguistic processing. *Cortex,* 8: 427-443.

Atkins, C. (1998, April). A treatment plan with real vision. ADVANCE for Occupational Therapists, p. 6).

Benson, F. D. and Ardila, A. (1996). *Aphasia: A clinical perspective.* New York: Oxford University Press.

Campbell, J. (1982). *Grammatical man: Information, entropy, language, and life.* New York: Simon and Schuster.

Cambier, J., Signoret, J.L., and Bolgert, F. (1989). Visual object agnosia: Current conceptions. *Rev Neurol (Paris),* 145 (8-9): 640-645.

Chusid, J. (1973). *Correlative neuroanatomy & functional neurology* (15th ed.). Los Altos, Calif.: LANGE Medical Publications.

Davis, G.A. (2007). *Aphasiology: Disorders and clinical practice* (2nd ed.) Boston: Pearson, Allyn and Bacon.

Eisenson, J. (1984). *Adult aphasia* (2nd ed.). Englewood Cliffs, N.J.: Prentice-Hall.

Gerstmann, J. (1940). Syndrome of finger agnosia, disorientation for right and left, agraphia, and acalculia. *Archives of Neurology and Psychiatry,* 44, 398-408.

Goss, B. (1982). *Processing communication.* Belmont, CA.: Wadsworth.

Head, H. (1926). *Aphasia and kindred disorders of speech.* New York: Cambridge University Press and Macmillian. (Reprinted in 1963 by Hafner Publishing Co., New York).

Hicks, S. and Sales, B. (2006). *Criminal profiling: Developing an effective science and practice*. Washington, D.C.: American Psychological Association.

Hillis, A. E. (2001). Cognitive neuropsychological approaches to rehabilitation of language disorders: Introduction. In *Language intervention in aphasia and related neurogenic communication disorders* (4th ed.). R. Chapey (Ed). Philadelphia: Lippincott Williams and Wilkins.

Kent, R. D. (1997). *The speech sciences*. San Diego: Singular Publishing Group.

Liberman, A. M. and Mattingly, I.G. (1985). The motor theory of speech perception revised. *Cognition*, 21: 1-36.

Lissauer, H. (1890). Ein Fall vol Seelenblindheit nebst einem Beitrag zur Theorie derselben [A case of visual agnosia with a contribution to theory]. *Archiv fur Psychiatrie*, 21, 222-270. Translated in Shallice, T., & Jackson, M. (1988). Lissauer on agnosia. *Cognitive Neuropsychology*, 5, 153-192.

Love, R. J. And Webb, W.G. (1996). *Neurology for the speech-language pathologist* (3rd ed.). Boston: Butterworth-Heinemann.

Luria, A. (1958). Brain disorders and language analysis. *Language and speech*, 1: 14-34.

Luria, A. (1964). Factors and Forms of Aphasia. In *Disorders of language*. A. DeReuck and M. O'Connor (Eds). London: J. & A. Churchill

Luria, A. (1966). *Higher cortical function in man*. New York: Basic Books.

Luria, A. (1970). *Traumatic aphasia: Its syndromes, psychology and treatment*. The Hague: Mouton.

Luria, A. (1974). Language and brain. *Brain and Language*, 1: 1-14.

Martin, F. (1997). *Introduction to audiology* (6th ed.). Boston: Allyn & Bacon.

McFarland, H.R. and Fortin, D. (1982). Amusia due to right temporoparietal infarct. Archives of Neurology, Vol. 39, No. 11: 725-727.

Nadeau, S.E. and Rothi, L.J. (2001). Rehabilitation of subcortical aphasia. In *Language intervention in aphasia and related neurogenic communication disorders* (4th ed.). R. Chapey (Ed). Philadelphia: Lippincott Williams and Wilkins.

Nicolosi, L., Harryman, E., and Kresheck, J. (1996). *Terminology of communication disorders: Speech-language-hearing* (4th ed.). Philadelphia: Lippincott Williams & Wilkins.

Odell, K., McNeil, M., Rosenbek, J., and Hunter, L. (1991). Perceptual characteristics of vowel and prosody production in apraxic, aphasic, and dysarthric speakers. *Journal of Speech and Hearing Research*, 34: 67-80.

Patterson, K. and Behrmann, M. (1997). Frequency and consistency effects in a pure surface dyslexic patient. *Journal of Experimental Psychology: Human Perception and Performance*, Vol. 23, No. 4: 1217-1231.

Raymer, A.M. and Rothi, L.J. (2001). Cognitive approaches to impairments of word comprehension and production. In *Language intervention in aphasia and related neurogenic communication disorders* (4th ed.). R. Chapey (Ed). Philadelphia: Lippincott Williams and Wilkins.

Schwartz, R.G. (2002). Phonological disorders. In *Human communication disorders: An introduction* (6th ed.). G. H. Shames and N. B. Anderson (Eds). Boston: Allyn & Bacon.

Sternberg, R. and Ben-Zeev, T. (2001). *Complex cognition: The psychology of human thought.* New York: Oxford University Press.

Tanner, D. (2006). An advanced course in communication sciences and disorders. San Diego: Plural.

Tanner, D. (2007). Redefining Wernicke's area: Receptive language and discourse semantics. *J Allied Health, 36, 63-66.*

Winner, E. And Karolyi, C. (1998). Artistry and aphasia. In *Acquired aphasia* (3rd ed.). M. Sarno (Ed). San Diego: Academic Press.

Zemlin, W.R. (1998). *Speech and hearing science: Anatomy and physiology.* Boston: Allyn and Bacon.

Chapter 5: Motor Speech Programming Disorders

"The greatest enemy of knowledge is not
ignorance, it is the illusion of knowledge."

Stephen William Hawking

Chapter Preview: This chapter addresses the three primary
components of high-level motor speech production: conceptualization,
formulation, and execution. Apraxia of speech, the impaired ability
to produce voluntary neuromuscular speech movements is discussed
including variations of this speech pathology: ideational, verbal, and
ideomotor apraxias. In addition, oral and limb apraxias are reviewed.
The Sequentially Ordered-Closed Loop Model of Apraxia of Speech
is described. There is a review of efficacy of apraxia of speech therapy
and a discussion of principles of evaluation and treatment.

Apraxia of Speech: The Tangled Tongue

Apraxia, *Greek* for inaction, was coined by the German psychiatrist
Hugo Liepmann. Although there are many historical references to
apraxic behaviors, Liepmann (1900) formally defined apraxia as an
inability to perform voluntary movements not due to paralysis or other
muscle tone pathologies. According to Buckingham, (1998, p. 269):
"The term has been used, often with qualifying modifier to describe
syndromes or parts of syndromes. The different conceptualizations of

apraxia in general have engendered inconsistencies for the definition of apraxia of speech." In this text, apraxia of speech is used as an all-encompassing term for the varieties of motor speech programming disorders.

Unlike aphasia, *apraxia of speech* is neither an expressive nor receptive language disorder; it is a breakdown in the ability to conceptualize, program, and execute the motor actions necessary to produce speech. Rarely does apraxia of speech occur independently of expressive aphasia, and when it does, it is usually mild; pure severe apraxia of speech is unusual. In addition, of the five basic *motor speech processes* of *respiration, phonation, articulation, resonance,* and *prosody,* apraxia of speech usually primarily affects articulation leaving the other processes less impaired. As such, apraxia of speech can be considered a nonsymbolic neurogenic communication disorder essentially involving the articulatory mechanism. Basically, apraxia of speech involves the patient knowing what he or she wants to say, but cannot motorically produce speech (in the absence of paralysis). In the most elemental of terms, aphasia is *amnesia for words* and apraxia of speech is a *tangled tongue.* As noted in Chapter 3, in the traditional definition of Broca's aphasia, apraxia of speech is a primary component along with expressive language disturbances. Apraxia of speech is characterized by struggled attempts to make voluntary utterances and consequently, it is one of the most frustrating communication disorders. For clinicians, it is also one of the most difficult to treat. There are three levels of motor speech organization: *conceptualization, formulation,* and *execution* with corresponding apraxias of speech: *ideational, verbal,* and *ideomotor.*

Overview of Motor Speech Organization and Apraxia of Speech

Neurological and cognitive theories of motor speech organization and disorders are many, varied, complex, and controversial. It is understandable that these theories are such for they address transforming processes of the mind, thoughts, to physical manifestations, voluntary speech acts. While it is true that mind-to-physical manifestations occur with other bodily functions such as walking and pointing for example, ideation to voluntary speech acts represents pure thought-to-movement transformations. This concept has significant philosophical implications and lies at the heart of human self-determination. As such, theories abound about this complex process with no consensus in sight.

Historically, John Hughlings Jackson (1878) and Aleksandr R. Luria (1974, 1970, 1966, 1964, 1958) addressed the manner in which ideas are transformed to movement and postulated several ways the process breaks down in neurological injury. To further complicate this issue, Jackson, Luria, and current neuroscientists have ventured down the localization road attempting to isolate the site of lesion causing this "ideation-to-kinetic" transformation breakdown (Buckingham, 1998). Ferrand (2007) considers the motor cortex to be inclusive of the primary, premotor, and supplementary motor areas. According to Wise, Greene, Büchel, and Scott (1999), the articulatory plan may be formulated in several areas of the brain besides Broca's area including the anterior insula and lateral premotor cortex. Because of the interconnection of brain sites and tracts, and because the brain operates holistically, as a practical rule, verbal apraxia typically can affect more or less, all three levels, of neurological motor speech organization.

Modern theories about motor speech organization propose that there are three apraxias of speech based on the level of motor speech organization: *ideational, verbal,* and *ideomotor.* As Table 5.1 shows, at the conceptual level, *ideational* apraxia of speech interrupts integration of the speech act into the concept. There is a disconnection between the idea and the motor plan to express it. According to Darley, Aronson, and Brown (1975), damage to cortical and subcortical structures cause disorders at the conceptual level. At the *formulation* level, verbal apraxia interrupts the formulation for the specific motor plan, i.e., voluntary speech acts. At the *execution* level, ideomotor apraxia of speech results in the impaired integration and sequencing of voluntary speech acts.

Table 5.1: Levels of Neurological Impairments and Apraxia of Speech

Neurological Level	Apraxia of Speech	Manifestations	Possible Primary Site(s) of Lesion
Conceptual	Ideational	Difficulty integrating the speech intention into the concept	Cortical and subcortical areas of the brain.
Formulation	Verbal	Impairments programming the motor plan for voluntary speech acts	Broca's area (left inferior frontal gyrus), anterior insula and lateral premotor cortex.
Execution	Ideomotor	Impaired integration and sequencing of voluntary speech movements	Broca's area proper and adjacent/ descending tracts.

Conceptualization of Motor Speech Acts

"The conceptual-programming stage represents the highest level of motor organization" (Duffy, 1995, p. 53). The conceptualization stage of motor speech organization involves all aspects of language but particularly *semantics* which is the fundamental meaning carried by a language code. The boundaries between symbolic language and motor speech production are indistinct when addressing the conceptualization stage of motor speech organization. However, the symbol-referent relationship, which is fundamental to semantics, is the cornerstone to it and drives motor speech production at the *morpheme, proposition,* and *discourse* levels. Embedded within utterances at each level are the neuromuscular requirements necessary to produce speech. Varley and Whiteside (2001) propose that apraxia of speech is the result of the speaker being unable to access stored movement plans and thus programming them anew. They suggest that many of the observable struggle behaviors common in apraxia of speech are the result of the speaker assembling and programming the utterance "online." It is at the conceptualization stage of motor speech organization where abstract thoughts are organized as motor speech intentions for eventual production. British neurologist, Macdonald Critchley (1970, 1964) likened this conceptual stage to the silent thinking process of the *preverbitum.*

> "Deficits in conceptualization often reflect diffuse impairment of cognitive or affective functions and are commonly associated with dementia, confusion, or other disturbances" (Duffy, 1995, p. 54).

At the most elemental conceptualization level, the spoken utterance consists of the morpheme and the neuromuscular organization to produce it. Each spoken morpheme, the smallest unit of meaning, is a phoneme or a collection of phonemes constituting the spoken symbol. This phoneme, or series of phonemes, is cognitively associated with the speaker's learned referents. A referent is that to which the symbol refers, i.e., people, objects, emotions, thoughts, and other aspects of reality. The conceptualization of the motor plan to produce a morpheme involves the phoneme or series of phonemes spoken to represent the ideational intent of the referent. This symbol-referent association is learned and modified over time. At the morpheme level of conceptualization, the motor speech requirements necessary to produce this basic unit of semantic meaning are generally organized for voluntary utterances.

The second level of conceptualization organization occurs with the proposition. As John Hughlings Jackson (1878) observed, speaking is more than uttering words; the basic unit of meaningful speech is the proposition. The proposition is the psychological intent of the utterance and the idea behind that which is spoken. As such, speakers organize speech at the conceptual propositional level where the general motor speech requirements necessary to express an idea are created and they are based the psychological intent driving it.

The third level of conceptualization occurs at the discourse semantic level. According to Sternberg and Ben-Zeev (2001), discourses are communicative units of language larger than individual sentences, and include conversations, lectures, stories, essays, and so forth. The discourse communicative intention is organized so it can be motorically programmed for speech. The concept driving the speech act is generally organized as a series of motor events that can enable motor speech discourse production.

Formulation of Motor Speech Acts

As discussed below, Karl Lashley's (1951) theory of motor speech production as "serially-ordered behaviors" serves as the basis for understanding the formulation level. Lashley proposed a "priming of expressive units" of speech production prior to their execution. This process lies between the conceptualization and execution stages of motor speech planning. Kent (1997, p. 304) summarizes the process: "In brief, to speak out a thought, first we need to hold the thought as a governing superstructure for behavior; second, we select and activate the units that will be used in expressing the thought as a spoken message; and, third, we put the activated units into the intended sequence." Formulation of motor speech involves selection of the individual speech behaviors necessary to the expression of the concept. The timing, speed, strength, and precision of muscular movements are formulated for the five basic motor speech processes: respiration, phonation, articulation, resonance, and prosody. Darley, Aronson, and Brown (1975) observe that the motor speech plan is integrally tied to body spatial-temporal factors and the speaker's body scheme.

> Apraxia of speech is sometimes associated with poor auditory discrimination abilities.

The speaker's respiratory support provides the foundation for all motor speech formulation. Phonation, articulation, resonance, and prosodic formulation variables are dependent on the patient's available air support for each utterance. For a given speech act, the timing, speed, strength, and precision of respiratory muscles are programmed to effect the compression of air to be used for speech production. The anticipated length, loudness, rate, and other variables related to respiratory support are integrated into the respiratory plan for a particular utterance. At the phonation level, voicing and voice onset temporal factors, pitch, loudness, and other variable are programmed, and of course, are also tied to respiratory support. Individual phonemes and their muscular timing, speed, strength, and precision for production are also programmed at the articulatory level. Velar valving is programmed as a binary function, i.e., off-on, for each individual phoneme and the appropriate nasalization. General prosodic factors for dynamic speech are also programmed. Essentially, at the formulation level of motor speech production, all of the neuromuscular requirements necessary to produce individual and connected phonemes are planned for a particular voluntary speech act. Duffy (1995, p. 55) summarizes the requirements and goals of motor speech formulation:

> Speech programming involves translation of the abstract linguistic-phonologic representation into a code that can be used by the motor system to generate movements that result in speech. This requires the selection of movements and the programming of their sequential and durational properties. More basically, the process must account for: identification of muscles, sequences for muscle contraction and relaxation; speed, strength, and duration of muscle excitation and inhibition; and coordination of speech muscle activities with other muscles involved in the act.

Integral to the formulation of utterances are adjustments for dynamic speech: *anticipatory* and *backward coarticulation* features. According to Ferrand (2007), anticipatory coarticulation occurs when a preceding phoneme modifies an ensuing one and vice versa for backward coarticulation, e.g., an upcoming phoneme influences a preceding one.

> Overshooting of an articulatory target is called an *anticipatory error* and undershooting is referred to a *perseveratory* one.

Execution of Motor Speech Plans

There is overlap between the execution of the motor speech program and upper motor neuron activation of speech muscles for the production of the individual phonemes. Consequently, the dividing line between motor speech plan execution and upper motor neuron activation is indistinct. Concerning speech pathologies, neither is there a clear distinction between the motor speech plan execution disorder, ideomotor apraxia of speech, and the upper motor neuron activation impairment, spastic dysarthria. Anatomically, the lesion or lesions resulting in motor speech plan execution disorders lie between Broca's area proper, i.e., smallest area exclusively controlling motor speech, and the motor strip and associated corticobulbar tracts. Execution of the motor speech plan involves integration and sequencing of voluntary speech movements related to the speaker's intention which are activated by adjacent descending upper motor neurons. Darley, Aronson, and Brown (1975, p. 63) summarize the relationship of the preprogrammed speech units and activation of the upper motor neuron system in the required temporal order: "The preprogrammed parcels are conceived of as activating the upper motor neuron system of both hemispheres with specific motor orders that lead to the performance of the behavioral acts."

Ideational Apraxia of Speech

As reported above, ideational apraxia of speech is a disruption of the ability to conceptualize motor speech acts; the gestalt of the idea and the speech movements required to express it are lost. *Conceptual apraxia* and ideational apraxia are terms sometimes used synonymously. According to Love and Webb (2001, p. 236), ideational apraxia is an impairment in the ability to carry out a hierarchical complex motor plan: "In ideational apraxia, individual movements can be called up, but a complex motor plan involving all elements of a motor act cannot successfully be executed." They note that ideational apraxia is often seen in bilateral lesions of the brain and generalized intellectual deterioration.

Ideational apraxia of speech, as in all apraxias, involves disturbances in the temporal and spatial sequencing of movements. In most cases however, the patient may be able to produce the individual units of the intended utterance but without connection to the concept driving them. There appears to be a loss of will to construct the series of speech movements to utter a concept. Many patients with ideational apraxia of speech display *speech abulia*, a loss of initiative and motivation to engage in voluntary social interaction. Patients with severe ideational apraxia of speech often resort to *echolalia* and the rote repetition of the last utterance spoken. Using echolalia, patients can engage in speech production giving the impression of wholeness and psychological integrity. Most notably in ideational apraxia of speech is the patient's lack of will to express a concept due to the complexities involved in connecting ideas to the necessary sequential motor speech acts. As noted above, ideational apraxia of speech may be seen in dementia, bilateral lesions of the brain, but especially in frontal lobe syndrome and disorders that affect dopamine and other neurotransmitter levels. Love and Webb (2001) observe that patients with ideational apraxia have serious survival issues due to their inability to manipulate the environment.

> Many treatments for Broca's aphasia also incorporate therapies for apraxia of speech.

Verbal Apraxia

Because verbal apraxia is a highly variable disorder, it is difficult to categorize and catalog its core behaviors and characteristics. A particular patient with verbal apraxia may present with speech pathologies differently from one speech act to the next. Additionally, patients with similar diagnoses can produce a wide variety of speech symptoms. Categorizing and cataloguing the core behaviors and characteristics of verbal apraxia is further complicated by the disparate symptoms seen in mild, moderate, and severe cases of the disorder. However, there are commonalities in the speech pathologies in patients with verbal apraxia and generalities can be drawn about this neurogenic communication disorder.

Buckingham (1998, p. 285) catalogs the typical phonetic aberrations in patients with verbal apraxia:

1. Awkward phonetic modulations of vowels and consonants (distortions);
2. Syllable stress errors and equalization of stress, which in turn affects any phonological process that is sensitive to stress, such as vowel reduction and flapping;
3. Initiating articulation and delayed verbal response times;
4. Smooth transition from one sound to the next;
5. Abnormal elongation of fricative and sonorant consonants;
6. Abnormal stopgap durations;
7. Abnormally lengthened vowels, syllables, and CV units;
8. Amplitude and fundamental frequency abnormalities;
9. Asynchronies and uncoupling of upper and lower articulatory systems that affect proper voice-onset time (VOT) parameters and oro/nasal productions;
10. Overly long intersegmental durations;
11. Difficulty adjusting rate of speech.

Duffy (2005) notes that consonant clusters are more frequently in error than singletons, and that error rates are higher for nonsense syllables and words than for meaningful sounds.

Darley, Aronson, and Brown (1975, p. 250), provide a classic example of mild to moderate verbal apraxia. It is called the "Tornado Man" passage, a recording of a patient describing a family fleeing from a tornado, and represents relatively pure verbal apraxia:

> I am looking <u>an</u> a drawing or <u>a-a pec-</u>picture of what is apparently a <u>tor-nuh-ner-nor-tornatiuhd blew-</u>brewing in the <u>c-c</u>ountry side. This is having an <u>nuh-nuh</u>mediate and frightening <u>ef-f-ff-fuh-feck</u> on a <u>fairm</u> fam<u>er</u>ly num<u>-ber-ing</u>—six uh humans and <u>af-ff-sss-uh-sh-suh-sorted</u> farm uh animals. <u>There</u> are quick-<u>uh-ly</u> going into <u>a-a sss-sor-</u>

<u>sormb</u> uh cellar with fright in their <u>ar-uh-eyes</u> and in their every-movement. "

According to Wambaugh, Duffy, McNeil, Robin, and Rogers (2006), the primary clinical characteristics of verbal apraxia include slow rate of speech, speech sound distortions and substitutions, and prosodic abnormalities. In addition, the errors in verbal apraxia are relatively consistent in terms of manner and place of production. Darley, Aronson, and Brown (1975) provide a detailed review of the clinical features of verbal apraxia including behavioral characteristics, factors influencing and not influencing apraxic speech behaviors, and associated features.

> The hallmark of apraxia of speech, like stuttering, is struggle during the speech act.

According to Darley, Aronson, and Brown (1975), apraxic patients effortfully grope to find the correct articulatory postures and sequences of phoneme production. These articulatory errors involve consonants more than vowels. The articulatory errors are complications of the act of articulation, i.e., substitutions, additions, repetitions, and prolongations and are close approximations to the target speech sounds. The schwa vowel may be present, and errors may be inconsistently anticipatory and perseverative. Apraxic patients typically can recognize their articulatory errors.

Darley, Aronson, and Brown (1975) note that articulatory errors increase with longer words and as the complexity of motor adjustments increase, initial consonants tend to be misarticulated more often than final ones, and high frequency phonemes are more accurately spoken. Automatic and reactive utterances are generally produced better than volitional-purposeful and spontaneous speech. Articulatory errors increase in apraxia of speech as the semantic significance and propositionality of the utterances increase and they decrease when correct auditory and visual models are provided. Repeated trials facilitate correct production more than repeated stimuli presentations. Table 5.2 summarizes the symptoms of verbal apraxia.

Table 5.2: Clinical Characteristics of Apraxia of Speech

Motor Speech Process	Characteristics
Prosody	Slow rate of speech Abnormal stop gaps Syllable stress errors Overly long intersegmental durations Difficulty adjusting rate of speech Abnormally lengthened vowels, syllables, and consonant-vowel units

Articulation	Complication errors:
	    Substitutions
	    Additions (schwa vowel)
	    Repetitions
	    Prolongations
	Errors more frequent on:
	    Consonants and consonant clusters
	    Initial phonemes
	    Low frequency phonemes
	    Phonemes require complex adjustments

Phonation-Resonance	Amplitude and fundamental frequency abnormalities Asynchronies and uncoupling of nasal and oral cavities Awkward modulation of vowels and consonants
Accessory and Related Features	Effortful groping (struggle) during speech More errors with increased semantic significance and propositionality Delayed verbal response time Automatic better than purposeful speech Errors inconsistently anticipatory or perseverative Self-recognition of errors Errors decrease with visual-auditory modeling

According to Darley, Aronson, and Brown (1975), the mental set of the apraxic patient does not affect his or her performance and neither does masking noise, delayed imitative responses, and the use of a mirror by the patient to monitor speech production. Oral apraxia, auditory perceptual disturbances, and oral sensation and perception impairments often co-occur with apraxia of speech.

Ideomotor Apraxia of Speech

As reported above, there is overlap between the execution of motor speech programs and upper motor neuron activation of speech muscles for individual phoneme production. Ideomotor apraxia of speech is a breakdown in the *execution* of the motor speech plan transmission to the upper motor neurons for *activation*. The likely site of lesion for ideomotor apraxia of speech includes Broca's area and adjacent descending neuronal tracts. As Darley, Aronson, and Brown (1975) observe, preprogrammed speech units activate the upper motor neuron system of both hemispheres. Consequently, patients with ideomotor apraxia of speech can present with apraxic speech and spastic dysarthria symptoms. Ideomotor apraxia of speech is common in global aphasia and brain damage secondary to major interruptions of the left middle cerebral artery. If patients are capable of producing speech, not only do they have the *complications* errors of verbal apraxia but also the *simplification* errors, distortions and omissions, of spastic dysarthria.

Primary Progressive, Oral, and Limb Apraxias

Primary progressive apraxia of speech is the gradual development of this motor speech disorder in the absence of generalized cognitive deficits. McNeil and Duffy (2001, p. 480) define primary progressive apraxia of speech (PPAOS):

> PPAOS can be defined tentatively as AOS of insidious onset, gradual progression, and prolonged course, in the absence of nonlanguage cognitive impairments, and sometimes in the absence of aphasia, for a substantial period of time or perpetually, due to a degenerative condition that presumably involves the left hemisphere's apparatus for translating the phonologic aspects of language into the learned kinetic parameters necessary for their expression through speech."

Primary progressive apraxia of speech is rare and is likely to co-occur in primary progressive aphasia (See Chapter 3). According to McNeil and Duffy (2001), there are only a small number of published case reports addressing this neurogenic communication disorder. However, the distinction between primary progressive aphasia and primary progressive apraxia of speech may be important for evaluation and treatment purposes.

Oral apraxia, similar to apraxia of speech, is the inability or impaired ability to purposefully perform nonspeech oral movements such as puckering, licking, and protruding the lips, smiling, biting the lower lip, lateralizing the tongue, and so forth. *Nonverbal oral apraxia, bucco-facial apraxia,* and *lingual apraxia* are terms sometimes used synonymously. This apraxia, like apraxia of speech, has the voluntary-involuntary dichotomy. As a result, oral nonspeech acts are impaired or impossible when the patient consciously and purposefully tries to perform them, but can be completed when little or no attention and thought are given to how they are done. According to Duffy (2005), apraxia of speech and oral apraxia frequently co-occur. However, there is not a 1:1 correlation relationship between the two and either one can exist in the absence of the other. Localizing the site or sites of lesion for oral apraxia have yielded disparate results. Duffy (2005) reports right lower face weakness, lingual weakness, and oral sensory deficits associated with nonverbal oral apraxia complaints in patients.

Limb apraxia, sometimes called *limb-kinetic apraxia*, is the patient's inability or impaired ability to use his or her body limbs to engage in purposeful movements. Like apraxia of speech and oral apraxia, patients with limb apraxia display the voluntary-involuntary dichotomy. For example during testing, limb apraxia may be present during pantomiming requests. If a patient with limb apraxia is asked to show how to light and smoke a cigarette, he or she may use the fingers, wrist, hand, and arm in such a way as to be unable to pantomime the required bodily functions sequentially. However, after the examination session is over, if the patient is a smoker, he or she can automatically complete the actions necessary to light and smoke a cigarette when little or no attention and thought are given to the necessary sequential limb actions. Similar limb apraxic behaviors can be observed with a toothbrush, key, eyeglasses, and so forth. Limb apraxia is often, but not exclusively, associated with left-hemisphere brain damage. According to Kaplan, Gallagher, and Glosser (1998), limb apraxia is difficult to distinguish from more basic pyramidal or extrapyramidal motor disorders and can be characterized as a general clumsiness.

> The patient's ability to sing familiar songs can be used to facilitate purposeful speech production.

Sequentially Ordered-Closed Loop Model of Apraxia of Speech

Plante and Beeson (2004) consider apraxia of speech to be primarily a phonetic disorder. However, more precisely, apraxia of speech is a subcategory of phonetic disorders, a disruption of *articulatory phonetics*. While it is acknowledged that apraxia of speech can disrupt all of the motor speech processes, it primarily affects articulation with respiration, phonation, resonance, and prosody affected secondarily and only as they pertain to general motor speech organization.

Miller (2000, p. 174), and others, have criticized the *central motor programming* theory of speech production advanced in the 1970s by Darley, Aronson, and Brown: "This perspective grew from models that envisaged separate levels succeeding each other in the genesis of word and speech production. A semantic lexicon fed forwards to a phonological lexicon, which added abstract specifications of sounds and their positions in an utterance. These in turn mapped on to motor commands, providing instructions for muscle movements to produce speech." The criticisms of the central programming theory involves the criteria by which speakers select articulatory parameters during speech acts and the self-perception of speech gesture targets. With regard to apraxia of speech, critics argue that the central programming breakdown theory simply does not adequately define the disorder nor does it distinguish apraxia of speech from other neurogenic communication disorders. According to Miller (2000) and others, central programming theory applied to apraxia of speech is at best incomplete and at worst totally flawed.

Although, several current models address the alleged weaknesses of the central programming theory such as feedback-feedforward, dynamic systems, connectionist, and target models (Ferrand, 2007), most are elaborations of theories proposed in the mid 1900s. Lashley's (1951) concept of *serially ordered speech behaviors* and Fairbank's (1954) speech mechanism as a *servosystem* provides the bases for a clinical model of apraxia of speech. These theories of motor speech planning and production can provide a foundation for the evaluation and treatment of apraxia of speech and meet the treatment guidelines proposed by Wambaugh, Duffy, McNeil, Robin, and Rogers (2006).

> Karl S. Lashley's famous article addressing brain engrams and learning was "Brain Mechanisms and Intelligence; A Quantitative Study of Injuries" published in The *American Journal of Psychology* in 1931.

Lashley's serially ordered speech behavior model addresses the temporal sequencing of neuromuscular actions involved in speech acts. The primary issue in serially ordered speech behaviors concerns which *elements* of speech are temporally serialized. It is beyond the scope of this book to address whether distinctive features, phonemes, syllables, words, grammatical structures or larger concepts such as propositions and intentions are the elements temporally serialized. These are controversial theories in neuroscience and a consensus is far from imminent. Suffice it to say that there are units of speech temporally serialized, selected in advance of an utterance, and at some neurological level, they are transformed into speech acts. Duffy (1995, p. 278) reports: "There is debate about whether AOS is a linguistic as opposed to a motor speech disorder. At this time, the weight of perceptual, acoustic, and physiologic evidence supports motor speech disorder explanations of AOS, in spite of the fact that AOS usually occurs in association with aphasia." Kent (1997) summarizes the serially ordered speech behavior model as consisting of three control mechanisms: *determining tendency, priming of expressive units,* and *schema of order.*

The determining tendency is the idea or notion that governs the whole organization of motor speech. It is related to the speaker's psychological intent to express a thought. This determining tendency is discussed above in the section on conceptualization of motor speech acts and it is proposed that the determining tendency occurs at the morpheme, proposition, and discourse levels. The psychological intent is organized for the eventual expression of a thought. The neurogenic communication disorder resulting from impairments at this level is ideational apraxia of speech.

The priming of expressive units involves the advanced selection of elements of speech for serialization. The selected units, be they distinctive features, phonemes, syllables, etc., are activated for eventual production during the speech act. As reported above, this process is the formulation of motor speech acts and verbal apraxia results from a breakdown at this level. Table 5.2 shows the primary prosodic, articulation, phonation-resonance, and accessory and related features of verbal apraxia.

The schema of order results in the selected elements activated in proper serial and temporal order. As noted above in the section addressing execution of motor speech plans, at this level there is initiation of the serially ordered sequence. A breakdown of this process results in ideomotor apraxia of speech and/or spastic dysarthria.

Motor speech organization, conceptualization, formulation, and execution, does not occur in the absence of feedback. Speech production is highly dependent on auditory and somesthetic feedback. The feedback is a closed loop system, a servo system (Fairbanks, 1954), where body and auditory sensations are looped back to the motor speech control center for evaluation and correction if necessary. As can be seen in Figure 5.1, in the closed loop system, muscles involved in respiration, phonation, articulation, and resonance receive commands from the controlling system to produce the movements required for the speech act. Respiratory muscles compress air and systematically relax and contract to allow the proper pressure and flow for speech production. Intrinsic and extrinsic laryngeal muscles modulate the airflow coming from the lungs for proper voice onset, pitch, and loudness. The articulatory muscles move rapidly from one articulatory position to another, and these articulatory gestures are of the required speed, strength, and trajectory to create the desired acoustic characteristics for intelligible speech. The muscles of the velopharyngeal mechanism connect and disconnect the oral and nasal cavities to effect the proper nasal resonance. All of the muscles of motor speech production interact with each other in a way that produces speech acts with a smooth rhythm and flow. Levet (1989) proposes a perceptual processing unit corresponding to Fairbank's programming system.

> Grant Fairbanks' groundbreaking article addressing the closed-loop model of speech production was, "A theory of the speech mechanism as a servosystem," published in the *Journal of Speech and Hearing Disorders* in 1954.

In the closed loop system, there is a hypothetical self-concept evaluator, part of the personality that monitors whether the speech act is within normal parameters. The self-concept evaluator receives ongoing auditory and somesthetic feedback about the speech act and makes judgments about its normalcy. The auditory feedback is received from both ears and includes air and bone conduction. The somesthetic feedback includes body sensations related to muscle strength, valve pressures, and trajectories of articulatory gestures. As long as the output falls within individually determined accuracy levels, i.e., the speech output is within a range of normal for the individual, the self-concept evaluator is not activated. However, if the speech act is flawed, and one or more aspects of its output are outside the range of normal for the speaker, the self-concept evaluator is activated and an error signal is sent to the central programmer for adjustment and correction. Consequently, compensatory neuromuscular adjustments are made to effect the necessary changes resulting in adjustment and correction in the ongoing speech act. If the adjustments and corrections are satisfactory, the speaker continues with new utterances. However, if they are insufficient, another error signal is sent to the central programmer, and more adjustments and corrections are made. In the closed loop feedback system, ongoing auditory and body feedback about speech production is evaluated for its normalcy, and adjustments and corrections are made as necessary.

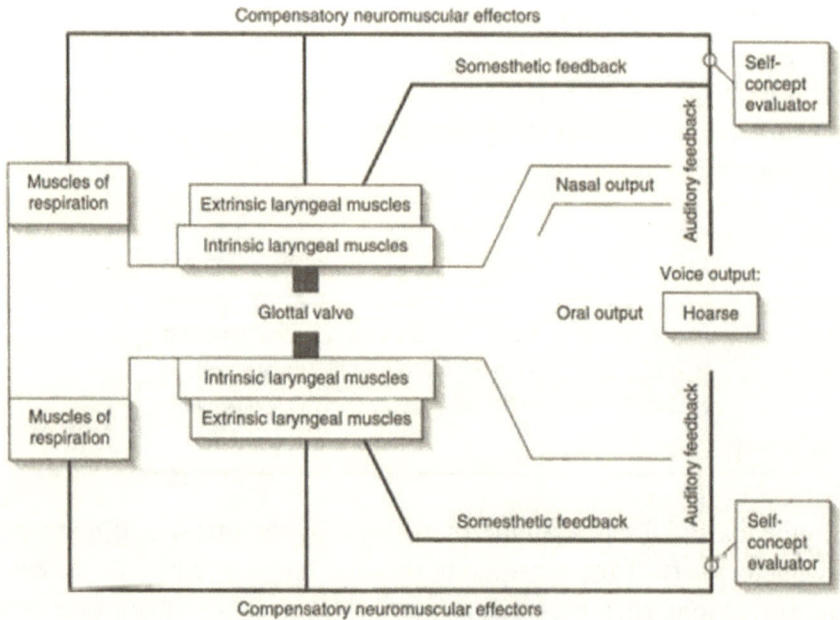

Figure 5.1: Sequentially Ordered-Closed Loop Model of Apraxia of Speech

In the Sequentially Ordered-Closed Loop Model of Apraxia of Speech, speech gestures are planned and activated by the central programmer and adjustments and corrections made during ongoing motor speech production based on closed loop feedback. In apraxia of speech, there is damage to the central programmer causing inaccurate sequentially ordered speech gestures. Duffy (1975, p. 265) found the following percentages of etiology of apraxia of speech: vascular (58%), degenerative (16%), traumatic (15%), tumor, left hemisphere (6%), other (5%), and multiple causes (1%). Of the vascular disturbances, single left hemisphere stroke accounted for nearly half of the vascular etiologies, 48% of the cases, and 10% were multiple strokes including the left hemisphere.

Certainly, there is a yet-to-be determined relationship between the linguistic and phonetic codes of the input signal and the central programmer's processing of them, but it is a disruption of the programmer per se that results in apraxia of speech. The central programmer is disrupted by neurological damage to the motor cortex and other brain sites discussed above. As a consequence of this neurological damage, inaccurate speech gesture commands are sent to the motor speech muscles. In mild cases of pure apraxia of speech, these speech gestures cause minimal speech errors and in severe cases, the patient is unable to produce voluntary speech. Duffy (2005) notes that in pure severe apraxia of speech, muteness may be present, but it rarely persists more than a few days. He also reports that severe apraxia of speech is usually accompanied by oral apraxia and automatic speech may not be better than volitional speech. Because of auditory and somesthetic feedback, in pure apraxia of speech, the patient is aware of the speech production errors. For those errors judged by the self-concept evaluator to be outside the acceptable tolerance range, compensatory adjustments are made at the source of the input to effect normalcy. Apraxia of speech results in disruptions of sequentially ordered motor speech commands which produce intolerable errors, and the articulatory complications, i.e., substitutions, additions, repetitions, prolongations, are compensatory actions taken by the patient to correct them.

Efficacy of Apraxia of Speech Treatment

The co-occurrence of aphasia is a negative prognostic factor in the treatment of apraxia of speech. According to Duffy (1995, p. 430), "Efficacy data and clinical impressions suggest that a variety of programs and techniques can be effective in managing AOS, especially when aphasia is not present or prominent." However, Rosenbek (1983) observes that when the apraxia of speech is more severe than the aphasia, i.e., Broca's aphasia with a preponderance of apraxia of speech (See Chapter 3), a high percentage regained some functional communication. Wertz (1984) reports that patients with apraxia of speech respond better to treatment addressing motor speech functions rather than language stimulation. Square, Martin, and Bose (2001) summarize traditional treatment approaches for patients with apraxia of speech by degrees of severity. For severely involved patients, treatment involves postural shaping and/or production of functional units of speech. Patients with mild and moderately severe apraxia of speech require rate and melodic flow treatments.

> Masking noise, positive instructional sets, and distractions do not appear to improve the speech production of patients with apraxia of speech.

Principles of Apraxia of Speech Evaluation and Treatment

Principle 1: An initial apraxia of speech screening and quick assessment should be conducted rather than a comprehensive diagnostic test.

As discussed in Chapter 3, the clinical practice of conducting one detailed and comprehensive aphasia evaluation before initiating treatment is theoretically flawed and outdated. Darley (1982), and others, note that longitudinal studies show that patients significantly evolve in type and severity of neurogenic communication disorder overtime. Further, medications may also affect the patient's presentation of symptoms. Additionally, apraxia of speech is often a temporary manifestation of stroke particularly in patients with increased cranial pressure and brain scans showing midline shifts. Because apraxia of speech is likely to co-occur with aphasic verbal encoding disorders, an initial apraxia of speech screening and quick assessment should be conducted as part of the aphasia assessment rather than an exhaustive test to be used as a primary measure of the disorder. Because of the fluctuating nature of apraxia of speech symptoms, a brief initial screening test should be administered during the initial bedside evaluation, and therapeutic evaluation should be ongoing and integral to each session.

Principle 2: General increasing of demands for volitional speech production and imitative tasks will distinguish apraxia of speech from other neurogenic communication disorders.

Duffy (2005) notes that imitative tasks and placing demands on the volitional sequencing of speech are likely to elicit the salient and distinguishing features of apraxia of speech. Imitative tasks and increased demands on volitional sequencing should begin with repetitions of vowels, continuants, plosive/affricates, diphthongs, and with a gradual increase to one, two, and three syllable words. Increased complexity of utterances can be obtained by imitative speech samples using one, two, and three syllable words and multiple word repetitions. Multiple repetitions and progressively longer words and phrases can detect mild apraxia of speech. Awareness of errors, struggle, and self-correction are noted with each speech sample.

Tanner and Culbertson (1999) suggest using a modified Likert scale to assess the patient's performance with communication abilities subjectively rated on a 1 (clearly abnormal or nonfunctional) to 5 (clearly normal or functional) continuum to screen for apraxia of speech. This quick assessment and other screening devices can give the clinician adequate information to begin diagnostic therapy.

Principle 3: An initial oral apraxia screening and quick assessment should be conducted in every case of suspected apraxia of speech.

The presence or absence of co-occurring oral apraxia can have therapeutic implications in the treatment of apraxia of speech. Patients with apraxia of speech who can engage in nonverbal purposeful oral motor movements can use this ability to prompt volitional speech behaviors. Consequently, patients should be tested to learn their capabilities purposefully to blow air from the lungs, smile, bite, and also engage in nonspeech lingual mobility behaviors such as protrusion, retraction, lateralization, depression, and elevation.

Principle 4: The treatment of ideational apraxia of speech involves integrating the speaker's concepts with the hierarchical complex motor plans to utter them.

Patients with ideational apraxia of speech suffer from various types and degrees of generalized intellectual impairments. As a result, many of these patients may not be able to profit from therapeutic experiences. For patients with the ability to profit from therapeutic experiences, the goal of ideational apraxia of speech treatment is to organize ongoing thoughts for expression. Treatment programs for this cognitive-motor speech planning disorder involve motivating the patient to construct speech acts of gradually increasing lengths. Sentence expansion drills, where the patient sequentially produces one, two, and three or more word utterances can be used to connect thoughts with the motor speech requirements to express them. For patients who are echolalic, topic shifting exercises can improve cognitive-motor speech planning abilities. Because ideational apraxia of speech can significantly affect the patient's functional communication, and thus quality of life, stimuli used for therapeutic drills and exercises should be important and functional to meet his or her basic wants and needs.

Principle 5: The treatment of verbal apraxia involves volitional formulation of the timing, speed, strength, and precision of muscular movements necessary to produce speech acts.

Behavioral management is at the heart of the treatment for apraxia of speech. Darley, Aronson, and Brown (1975, p. 279) observe: "The goal of therapy is to help the apraxic patient regain voluntary accurate control in programming the position of his articulators to produce phonemes and phoneme sequences." Regarding behavioral management approaches in the treatment of verbal apraxia, Duffy (1995, p. 423) notes: "They all share an emphasis on careful stimulus selection, an orderly progression of treatment tasks, and the use of intensive and systematic drill."

The goal of verbal apraxia therapy is to move the patient from volitional motor speech construction of single articulatory gestures to more complex speech acts. For patients with severe verbal apraxia, the goal may be to produce simple respiratory, phonatory, and articulatory muscle movements or action necessary for basic speech acts. For example, a simple respiratory action might be to push air through the oral tract consciously and purposefully. Using behavioral management procedures and techniques, the patient gradually learns to voluntarily produce simple, noncomplex muscle movements and actions. The progression of speech-related tasks includes vowels, continuants, plosive/affricates, diphthongs, multiple syllables, short words, longer words, phrases, and discourse. Operant conditioning, using rewards for gradual improvement of motor speech behaviors, is the best behavioral management approach. The treatment involves immediate rewarding of desired behaviors, or close approximations to them, cues and prompts, and the use of schedules of reinforcement.

> Visual biofeedback regarding tongue movements is a helpful therapy in treating apraxia of speech (Katz, Bharadwaj, and Carstens, 1999).

Principle 6: The treatment of ideomotor apraxia of speech involves execution of motor speech plans and neuromuscular therapies.

Because there is often no clear distinction between execution of the motor speech program and the activation of upper motor neurons for the production of speech, combining programming and neuromuscular therapies is necessary. In addition, because ideomotor apraxia of speech often involves aphasic disturbances, it may be necessary to combine language, motor speech formulation, and spastic dysarthria therapies. Language goals involving wordfinding and sentence construction activities are combined with apraxic and spastic dysarthria treatment objectives. In severe cases of ideomotor apraxia of speech, objectives may be for the patient to produce approximations of several words and phrases which carry meaning for the patient, his or her family and friends, and rehabilitation staff. In mild cases of ideomotor apraxia of speech, the goal may be to reduce complication and simplification errors to improve speech intelligibility of utterances expressing basic wants and needs.

Principle 7: Patients who are aware of speech programming errors and also self-corrective can engage in self-therapeutic relearning of motor speech programming with each speech act.

Patients who are consistently aware of their motor speech programming errors and correct them without the benefit of a therapist, can in effect, engage in self-therapy with each utterance. Because their feedback mechanisms allow detection of speech production errors, they are cued to ongoing speech programming disruptions. When confronted with speech programming errors, the self-corrective patient can correct them using trial-and-error articulatory posturing. Consequently, the aware and self-corrective patient engages in self-therapy with each utterance effectively providing independent and continuous relearning with each speech act.

Principle 8: Using nonspeech oral prompts in patients without co-occurring oral apraxia can facilitate initiation of speech movements in patients with apraxia of speech.

Many patients with apraxia of speech retain the ability to make nonspeech oral and lingual movements. These patients can use the ability to make volitional nonspeech articulatory approximations to initiate speech acts. For example, a patient unable to make the /f/ phoneme to initiate speech in the production of the word "first," can consciously bite the lower lip to prompt the word. Drills using the nonspeech biting of the lower lip for articulation transition for words beginning with /f/ will facilitate initiation of speech acts. Other nonverbal oral and lingual movements for articulation transition include touching the tip of the tongue to the alveolar ridge, tongue protrusion, placing the tongue between the upper and lower teeth, and smiling.

Principle 9: Retained automatic speech abilities can be used to ease expression.

Darley, Aronson, and Brown (1975, p. 281) observe that patients with apraxia of speech can use automatic speech to facilitate expression: "One can run through a repertoire of familiar expressions that will probably be easy for the patient to say and will help him once again obtain the 'feel' of generating speech easily." Many patients can produce familiar songs and everyday expressions such as "hello," "thank you," and "goodbye" in complex contexts while being unable purposefully to produce the individual phonemes, syllables, and words. When possible, they should produce an automatic expression with additional words to expand the length of the speech act.

Principle 10: Optimal therapies for apraxia of speech facilitate motor speech programming and execution by using expansion exercises, completion drills, and melodic cues.

Three exercises are effective in improving motor speech programming and execution in apraxic patients: sentence expansion, phrase completion, and melodic intonation therapy (MIT). Sentence expansion drills have the patient expand his or her one and two-word utterances. For example, if a patient responds to the question, "How are you today?" with the limited expression "Fine," the clinician uses a verbal or visual prompt to expand the utterance. The patient is encouraged to say, "I am find today," or "Fine, thank you." By expanding the utterance, the patient purposefully connects the idea to an utterance, creates a more complex motor speech program, and activates it.

Phrase completion drills are appropriate for patients with little or no abilities to produce purposeful utterances. They involve the patient uttering a word in response to an incomplete phrase prompt, such as "Red, white, and _____," Please pass the _____," and "The United States of _____." Phrase completion exercises address speech initiation deficiencies as well as programming impairments.

Melodic intonation therapy (Sparks, Helm, and Albert, 1974) theoretically uses melodies originating from the right hemisphere of the brain to cue or prompt motor speech production in patients with expressive aphasia. Using melody and tapping to progressively longer syllable productions, the patient produces more complex voluntary utterances. Theoretically, music stimulates the right hemisphere of the brain thus facilitating naming and programming.

Figure 5.2 summarizes the principles of treatment for motor speech programming disorders.

An initial apraxia of speech screening and quick assessment should be conducted rather than a comprehensive diagnostic test.
General increasing of demands for volitional speech production and imitative tasks will distinguish apraxia of speech from other neurogenic communication disorders.
An initial oral apraxia screening and quick assessment should be conducted in every case of suspected apraxia of speech.
The treatment of ideational apraxia of speech involves integrating the speaker's concepts with the hierarchical complex motor plans to utter them.
The treatment of verbal apraxia involves volitional formulation of the timing, speed, strength, and precision of muscular movements necessary to produce speech acts.
The treatment of ideomotor apraxia of speech involves execution of motor speech plans and neuromuscular therapies.
Patients who are aware of speech programming errors and also self-corrective can engage in self-therapeutic relearning of motor speech programming with each speech act.
Using nonspeech oral prompts in patients without co-occurring oral apraxia can facilitate initiation of speech movements in patients with apraxia of speech.
Retained automatic speech abilities can be used to ease expression.
Optimal therapies for apraxia of speech facilitate motor speech programming and execution by using expansion exercises, completion drills, and melodic cues.
Formal behavioral management techniques are optimal treatment methods for apraxia of speech.

Figure 5.2: Principles of motor speech programming treatment.

Chapter Summary

Motor speech programming disorders involve high-level impairments in the ability to conceptualize, formulate, and execute speech acts. Motor speech programming can be viewed as a sequentially ordered-closed loop speech act and apraxia of speech results from a breakdown in the process. Ideational, verbal, and ideomotor apraxias are variations of these high-level motor speech production disorders.

Study and Discussion Questions

1. Compare and contrast apraxia of speech and Broca's aphasia.
2. List and describe the five basic motor speech processes.
3. What are the levels of the levels of motor speech conceptualization?
4. Describe anticipatory and backward coarticulation features.
5. Describe ideational apraxia of speech.
6. Describe verbal apraxia.
7. Describe ideomotor apraxia of speech.
8. Define and describe primary progressive, oral and limb apraxias.
9. What is the Sequentially Ordered-Closed Loop Model of Apraxia of Speech? Describe it as it relates to the various apraxias.
10. List and discuss the principles of apraxia of speech evaluation and treatment.

References

Buckingham, H. W. (1998). Explanations for the concept of apraxia of speech. In *Acquired aphasia* (3rd ed.). M. Sarno (Ed). San Diego: Academic Press.

Critchley, M. (1964). The neurology of psychotic speech. *British Journal of Psychiatry*, 110: 353-364.

Critchley, M. (1970). *Aphasiology and other aspects of language.* London: Edward Aronld.

Darley, F., Aronson, A., and Brown, J. (1975). *Motor speech disorders.* Philadelphia: W. B. Saunders.

Duffy, J. R. (1995). *Motor speech disorders: Substrates, differential diagnosis, and management.* St. Louis: Mosby.

Duffy, J.R. (2005). *Motor speech disorders: Substrates, differential diagnosis, and management* (2nd ed.). St. Louis: Mosby.

Fairbanks, G. (1954). Systematic research in experimental phonetics: A theory of the speech mechanism as a servosystem. *Journal of Speech and Hearing Disorders,* 19: 133-139.

Ferrand, C. T. (2007). *Speech sciences: An integrated approach to theory and clinical practice* (2nd ed.). Boston: Pearson Allyn & Bacon.

Jackson, J. (1878). On affections of speech from diseases of the brain. *Brain.* 1: 301-330.

Kaplan, E., Gallagher, R., and Glosser, G. (1998). Aphasia related disorders. In *Acquired aphasia* (3rd ed.). M. Sarno (Ed). San Diego: Academic Press.

Katz, W. F., Bharadwaj, S. V., & Carstens, B. (1999). Electromagnetic articulography treatment for an adult with Broca's aphasia and apraxia of speech. *Journal of Speech, Language, and Hearing Research, 42*: 1355-1366.

Kent, R. D. (1997). *The speech sciences.* San Diego: Singular Publishing Group.

Lashley, K. (1951). The problem of serial order in behavior. In J. A. Jeffress (Ed) *Cerebral mechanisms in behavior* (pp. 112-136). New York: Wiley.

Levelt, W. (1989). *Speaking: From intention to articulation.* Cambridge, MA: MIT Press.

Liepmann, H. (1900). Das Krankheitsbild der apraxie. *Monatsschrift Psychiatrie und Neurologie*, 8, 182-197.

Love, R. J. And Webb, W.G. (1996). *Neurology for the speech-language pathologist* (3rd ed.). Boston: Butterworth-Heinemann.

Love, R. J. And Webb, W.G. (2001). *Neurology for the speech-language pathologist* (4rd ed.). Boston: Butterworth-Heinemann.

Luria, A. (1958). Brain disorders and language analysis. *Language and speech,* 1: 14-34.

Luria, A. (1964). Factors and forms of aphasia. In *Disorders of language.* A. DeReuck and M. O'Connor (Eds). London: J. & A. Churchill.

Luria, A. (1966). *Higher cortical function in man.* New York: Basic Books.

Luria, A. (1970). *Traumatic aphasia: Its syndromes, psychology and treatment.* The Hague: Mouton.

Luria, A. (1974). Language and brain. *Brain and Language*, 1: 1-14.

McNeil, M. and Duffy, J. (2001). Primary progressive aphasia. . In *Language intervention in aphasia and related neurogenic communication disorders* (4th ed.). R. Chapey (Ed). Philadelphia: Lippincott Williams and Wilkins.

Miller, N. (2000). Changing ideas in apraxia of speech. In *Acquired neurogenic communication disorders: A clinical perspective.* I. Papathanasiou (Ed). London: Whurr.

Plante, E. and Beeson, P. (2004). *Communication and communication disorders: A clinical introduction* (2nd ed.). Boston: Pearson.

Rosenbek, J.C. (1983). Treatment for apraxia of speech in adults. In W. H. Perkins (Ed). *Dysarthria and apraxia.* New York: Thieme-Stratton.

Sparks, R.W., Helm, N. And Albert, M. (1974). Aphasia rehabilitation resulting from melodic intonation therapy. *Cortex* 10: 303-316.

Square, P., Martin, R., and Bose, A. (2001). Nature and treatment of neuromotor speech disorders in aphasia. In *Language intervention in aphasia and related neurogenic communication disorders* (4th ed.). R. Chapey (Ed). Philadelphia: Lippincott Williams and Wilkins.

Sternberg, R. and Ben-Zeev, T. (2001). *Complex cognition: The psychology of human thought.* New York: Oxford University Press.

Tanner, D. and Culbertson, W. (1999). *Quick assessment for apraxia of speech.* Oceanside, CA.: Academic Communication Associates.

Varley, R. and Whiteside, S. (2001). What is the underlying impairment in acquired apraxia of speech? Aphasiology, 15 (1), 39-84.

Wambaugh, J.L., Duffy, J.R., McNeil, M.R., Robin, D.A., and Rogers, M.A., (2006). Treatment guidelines for acquired apraxia of speech: A synthesis and evaluation of the evidence. *Journal of Medical Speech-Language Pathology*, Volume 14, Number 2, pp. xv-xxxiii.

Wertz, R. T. (1984). Response to treatment in patients with apraxia of speech. In J. Rosenbek, M. McNeil and A. Aronson (Eds). *Apraxia of speech: Physiology, acoustics, linguistic, management*. San Diego: College-Hill Press.

Wise, R.J.S., Greene, J., Büchel, C., and Scott, S.K. (1999). Brain regions involved in articulation. *Lancet*, 353: 1057-61.

Chapter Six: The Dysathrias

"Science is a way of thinking much
more than it is a body of knowledge."

Carl Sagan

Chapter Preview: This chapter examines the dysarthrias and
separates the individual impairments into paralytic, coordination,
and movement neuromuscular communication disorders. The
paralytic dysarthrias, flaccid, spastic, and unilateral upper motor
neuron disorders, are reviewed including the affected motor speech
processes and associated speech pathologies. In this chapter there
is also a review of ataxic dysarthria, a coordination neuromuscular
communication disorder. Hypokinetic and hyperkinetic (quick and
slow) dysarthrias are examined concerning the effects of movement
dysfunctions on motor speech production. Several mixed and multiple
dysarthrias causing diseases and disorders are also reviewed. The
value and efficacy of dysarthria treatments are discussed and there
are principles for optimal dysarthria therapies.

Dysarthria: The Paralyzed Tongue

When discussing motor speech disorders, in the most elemental
of terms, *apraxia of speech* is a "tangled tongue" and *dysarthria*
is a "paralyzed tongue." Dysarthria is a general category of
neurogenic communication disorders resulting from impairments of

neuromuscular control. When dysarthria completely eliminates the ability to communicate, the patient is *anarthric* while the *dysarthric* patient has a milder form of the disorder. However, in this book, dysarthria refers the partial or complete disruption in the ability to communicate due to neuromuscular impairments. Dysarthria occurs because of degrees of damage to the central or peripheral nervous system and can affect one, several, or all of the five basic *motor speech processes*: *respiration, phonation, articulation, resonance,* and *prosody.*

Overview of Motor Speech Physical Laws and Theories

As Table 6.1 shows, there are applicable physical laws and theories for each of the motor speech processes. Respiration provides the raw compressed air from which speech is formed. The primary function of respiration is to sustain life by providing the body with oxygen and removing carbon dioxide. The secondary function of respiration is to compress air and gradually expel it during speech production. The chest cavity expands allowing air to enter the lungs and by gradually decreasing the size of the cavity, air is expelled. The physical laws involved in respiration are *Boyle's Law* and the *Kinetic Theory of Gases* (Zemlin, 1998). Generally, these laws dictate that a given quantity of gas varies inversely with its pressure, and gas flows from a region of high to low pressure and vice versa. *Inspiration* is the taking of air into the lungs and *expiration* is the expelling of it. During expiration, the pressure in the lungs is greater than the atmospheric pressure, and the air flows outward through the speaker's mouth and nose where it is valved to produce speech sounds.

Table 6.1: Motor Speech Production Physical Laws and Theories

Motor Speech Processes	Physiological Function	Physical Laws and Theories
Respiration	Air Compression for Speech Production	Boyle's Law and the Kinetic Theory of Gases
Phonation	Energizing Speech for Speech Production	Myoelastic-Aerodynamic Principle of Voice Production
Articulation	Shaping Compressed Air for Speech Production	Serially-Ordered Speech Acts
Resonance	Nasal Coupling and Nasality During Speech Production	Double Helmholtz Resonator
Prosody	Speech Rhythm and Flow	Closed-Loop Feedback (Servosystem)

Phonation is the vibration of the vocal folds to produce speech sounds. Not all phonemes are voiced and those that differ only by the voicing distinctive feature are *cognates*. The vocal folds are capable of vibrating rapidly due to muscular elasticity and the Bernoulli principle, i.e., the *Myoelastic-Aerodynamic Principle of Vocal of Voice Production*. In women, the average rate of vocal cord vibration is approximately 250 cycles-per-second and in men, they vibrate, on average, about 130 times per second. The amplitude of vocal cord vibration gives the perception of loudness and the frequency of vibration is associated with pitch. However, the amplitude-loudness and frequency-pitch relationships, while positively correlated, are not linearly proportional, i.e., a 1:1 relationship. Quality of voice, whether it is breathy, harsh, hoarse, etc. is related to its spectral characteristics and the efficiency of vocal cord vibration. The sliding, rocking, and rotating action of the arytenoid cartilages, and movements by other laryngeal cartilages, muscles, and structures, loosened and tightened the vocal folds. Increase or decrease in the *mass/unit length* of the vocal folds is a primary factor in the pitch changing mechanism.

> The Bernoulli principle is the reason airplane wings have lift when moving through air.

The primary articulators are the lips, tongue, teeth, mandible, and palates (soft and hard). Articulation is the process of shaping the compressed air coming from the lungs so that speech sounds, *phonemes*, are produced. This is done by rapidly valving the airstream. Dynamic speech is usually done so rapidly that the articulators only approximate their ideal points of contacts. Consequently in ongoing speech, the phonemes preceding and following the target one affect the precision of articulatory points of contacts. The more rapid the speech production, the more phonemes become more like each other. This is the concept of *serially ordered speech events* and that dynamic speech is a *stream of articulatory gestures. Coarticulation* is the overlapping of movements during speech which leads to *assimilation*; the effect one phoneme has on another.

The speech resonating chamber, approximately 17 cm in length, is a *double Helmholtz system*. The configuration, length, size, and texture of the resonating chamber give speech sounds their distinctive acoustic qualities. The velopharyngeal port is where the velum (soft palate) contacts the nasopharynx and is an important speech valving site. While all phonemes have nasal resonance, when the velopharyngeal port is opened, there is an increase in nasal emission and resonance. When the velopharyngeal port is closed, there is a decrease in nasal emission and resonance. The velum operates on a binary function, e.g., on-off, regarding opening and closing of the velopharyngeal port.

Prosody is broadly defined as the fluency, cadence, melody, inflection, and rate of speech. It includes acoustic patterns of stress, intonation, pitch, and loudness variations. While the speaker's fluency is dependent on all aspects of motor speech production, feedback plays a fundamental role. Speech feedback is a closed-loop, *servosystem* where auditory and physical sensations about the speech act are sent to speaker for adjustment and correction should intolerable errors in production occur. The ongoing feedback, adjustments, and corrections play a major role in the overall fluency of a speaker.

> The triangular-shaped arytenoid cartilages of the larynx are critical in changing vocal cord tension and adjusting the mass per unit length of the vocal folds. In pitch adjustment, they "slide," "rock," and "rotate."

Categorizing Dysarthria

In the not-so-distant past, students in communication sciences and disorders studied a hodgepodge of neuromuscular communication disorders in "organics" and disease-based courses. Students learned about the speech characteristics of cerebral palsy, Parkinson's disease, muscular dystrophy, multiple sclerosis, and so forth in various apparently unrelated courses other than they addressed motor speech disorders. In 1975, Darley, Aronson, and Brown at the Mayo Clinic in Rochester, Minnesota set the foundation for a new way of viewing dysarthria with the publication of their book *Motor Speech Disorders*. They proposed that motor speech disorders be classified by the level of neurological deficits and identified *flaccid, spastic, ataxic, hypokinetic, hyperkinetic,* and *mixed dysarthrias.* This classification system remained essentially unchanged until Duffy (2005, 1995) included *unilateral upper motor neuron dysarthria* as a distinguishable motor speech disorder. As Table 6.2 shows, dysarthria can further be classified as *paralytic, coordination,* and *movement* dysarthrias to reflect differences in treatment objectives. While it is acknowledged that all dysarthrias involve paralytic, coordination, and movement symptoms affecting motor speech production, the primary treatment objectives differ between the categories.

Table 6.2: Paralytic, Coordination, and Movement Dysarthrias

Paralytic	Coordination	Movement
Flaccid	Ataxic	Hypokinetic
Spastic		Hyperkinetic Quick Slow
Unilateral Upper Motor Neuron		

Paralytic Dysarthrias

Paralysis is the complete loss of function for a specific muscle or a group of muscles. *Paresis* is partial, mild, or incomplete functional muscle impairment. When one or more of the motor speech production muscles are paralyzed, paralytic dysarthria results. The paralytic dysarthrias primarily involve increased or decreased tone of the motor speech production musculature. Three paralytic dysarthrias have been identified: flaccid, spastic, and unilateral upper motor neuron.

Flaccid Dysarthria

According to Duffy (2005), flaccid dysarthria accounts for 9.1% of all dysarthrias. Flaccid dysarthria is a disorder of the *lower motor neuron* system also known as the "final common pathway" because all motor movement impulses must travel it. There are four components to the lower motor neuron system: cell body and dendrites, axon, myoneural junction, and muscle fibers. Many diseases and disorder can damage the lower motor neuron system and any one of its four components. According to Haynes and Pindzola (2004, p. 259) "Flaccid dysarthrias result from disorders (or lesions) of the lower motor neuron system. The muscle-movement problem may be progressive, as in myasthenia gravis, or may affect the bulbar motor units, as in the bulbar palsies." Diminished reflexes, hypotonia (decreased muscle tone), and muscle weakness and atrophy are common symptoms of flaccid dysarthria. Damage to cranial nerves V (Trigeminal), X (Vagus), and XII (Hypoglossal) primarily result in flaccid dysarthria. The symptoms of flaccid dysarthria depend on the motor speech processes affected: respiration, phonation, articulation, resonance, and prosody.

As Table 6.3 shows, the speech pathologies in flaccid dysarthria can be categorized by the impaired motor speech process. The symptoms of flaccid dysarthria, and whether or not they affect a particular motor speech process, depend on the specific nerve or nerves damaged. When the respiratory motor speech process is affected in flaccid dysarthria, the patient is likely to have reduced vital capacity. Reduced respiratory support for speech production results in impaired expiratory control and reduced loudness. Phonatory impairments include voice quality abnormalities such as continuous breathiness or harshness, and monopitch and/or monoloudness. Because of weakness of the phonatory muscles, some patients also may have audible inspiration. As for articulation, the patient with flaccid dysarthria produces imprecise consonants, usually distortions. Hypernasality results from impaired velopharyngeal valving and the patient may also have audible nasal emission during speech. Primarily due to lack of respiratory support, the patient may also have disrupted rhythm of speech including short phrasing. Associated features of flaccid dysarthria include muscle fasciculation (twitching) and drooling.

Table 6.3: Motor Speech Processes and Speech Pathologies in Flaccid Dysarthria

Motor Speech Process	Motor Speech Pathologies
Respiration	Reduced Vital Capacity Reduced Loudness Impaired Expiratory Control
Phonation	Voice Quality Impairments (Continuous Breathiness or Harshness) Monotonous Pitch and/or Loudness Audible Inspiration
Articulation	Imprecise Consonant Production
Resonance	Hypernasality Nasal Emission
Prosody	Short Phrasing

> Palsy: Partial or complete paralysis; may be accompanied by shaking or tremor of the body.

Spastic Dysarthria

Spastic dysarthria occurs with about the same frequency as flaccid dysarthria (Duffy, 2005). Spastic dysarthria results from damage to the *upper motor neuron* system. The upper motor neuron system has both a direct and indirect route to the lower motor neuron system. The direct route is involved in fine motor movements and the indirect route, through the basal ganglia and reticular activation center of the brain stem, is responsible for posture and movement spatial orientation. Spastic muscles are weak and they have exaggerated stretch reflexes, reduced range of motion, increased tone, and produce slow bodily movements. Strokes and degenerative diseases are the most common causes of spastic dysarthria, although traumas, tumors, infections, and inflammatory conditions are also etiological factors.

Patients with bilateral damage to the upper motor neuron system may present with a variety of symptoms depending on the motor speech process affected (See Table 6.4). Because speech production is dependent on respiratory support, patients with spastic dysarthria often produce short utterances primarily due to increased muscle resistance. When phonation is affected, there are monoloudness and monopitch, the tendency to produce a low pitch with frequent pitch breaks, and a harsh, strained voice quality. Articulation is produced imprecisely and with frequent distortions of phonemes. Although patients with spastic dysarthria may produce phonemes in isolation with normal nasal resonance, during connected speech, hypernasality may be present. This is due to the slow closing of the velopharyngeal port during speech production. Patients with spastic dysarthria tend to produce speech slowly and with reduced stress.

Table 6.4: Motor Speech Processes and Speech Pathologies in Spastic Dysarthria

Motor Speech Process	Motor Speech Pathologies
Respiration	Short Phrasing
Phonation	Low Pitch Pitch Breaks Harsh Voice Quality Strained Phonation Monopitch Monoloudness
Articulation	Imprecise and Distorted Speech
Resonance	Assimilated Hypernasality
Prosody	Slow Rate of Speech Reduced Stress

Unilateral Upper Motor Neuron Dysarthria

"Unilateral upper motor neuron (UUMN) dysarthria is a distinguishable motor speech disorder that is associated with damage to the upper motor neurons (UMNs) that carry impulses to the cranial and spinal nerves that supply the speech muscles" (Duffy, 1995, p. 222). Duffy goes on to note that UUMN, in contrast to other dysarthria types, is an anatomic rather than pathophysiologic designation and it occurs at a rate comparable to that of other major single dysarthria types. This dysarthria can be caused by damage to the right or left upper motor neuron tracts with paresis or paralysis on the opposite of the side of the neurological damage.

Stroke is the most common cause of unilateral upper motor neuron dysarthria with more than 90% of the cases arising from vascular disturbances (Duffy and Folger, 1986). The primary clinical features of UUMN dysarthria include hemiplegia or hemiparesis, impaired skilled movements, central facial weakness at rest and during voluntary movement, and tongue weakness. There is also increased muscle tone, spasticity, clonus (muscle contractions due to sudden stretching), and hyperactive stretch reflexes.

According to Duffy (2005), the most pervasive speech impairment associated with unilateral upper motor neuron dysarthria is imprecise consonant production with irregular articulatory breakdowns. The irregular articulatory breakdowns may be related to general articulation imprecision seen in speech muscle weakness (Landau, 1988). According to Duffy (2005), 57% of patients with UUMN had phonatory deficits. Resonance disorders occurred in 14% of the cases. Prosodic disturbances include a slow rate of speech with an increased rate of speech occurring in some patients. Excess and equal stress are also symptoms of prosodic disruptions (See Table 6.5).

Table 6.5: Motor Speech Processes and Speech Pathologies in Unilateral Upper Motor Neuron Dysarthria

Motor Speech Process	Motor Speech Pathologies
Respiration	Negligible Impairment
Phonation	Harsh Voice Quality Decreased Loudness
Articulation	Imprecise Consonants Irregular Articulatory Breakdowns
Resonance	Hypernasility
Prosody	Slow Rate of Speech Increased Rate in Segments Excess and Equal Stress

According to Duffy (2005), unilateral upper motor neuron dysarthria is usually only mild to moderate in severity and the prognosis is often good.

Coordination Dysarthria

When dysarthria affects muscle tone, strength, rate of speech, and articulatory precision, the patient's ability to coordinate motor speech acts is impaired. Consequently, all dysarthrias, more or less, affect coordinated motor speech production abilities of the patient.

However, ataxic dysarthria is the primary coordination neuromuscular communication disorder directly resulting from damage to the cerebellar system.

Ataxic Dysarthria

Ataxic dysarthria results from generalized and bilateral damage to the cerebellum and the tracts leading to and from it. "The cerebellum is considered to function by imposing its control upon posture and movement that it does not initiate" (Darley, Aronson, and Brown, 1975, p. 59). The cerebellum is considered the "great modulator of muscular movement" in that it does not initiate movements, but coordinates them. Without the modulating function of the cerebellum, motor impulses would cause movements to be overactive, and result in overshooting of targets. The cerebellum inhibits gross functional muscle movements and is also involved with equilibrium. Specifically, the cerebellum influences the direction, timing, and force of movements. According to Duffy (2005), ataxic dysarthria is caused by degenerative diseases (35%), vascular damage (13%), demyelination (17%), undetermined factors (15%), toxic and metabolic disorders (5%), trauma (5%), inflammation (4%), tumors (3%), multiple causes (1%), and other (1%), e.g., depression and personality disorders.

The respiratory motor speech process is not often affected in ataxic dysarthria, but some patients, especially those with generalized and multiple causative factors, have altered smooth cycling of respiration. Voice quality disturbances usually involve harshness and are often accompanied by monotonous pitch and loudness. Patients with ataxic dysarthria typically produce imprecise, distorted consonants, prolong phonemes, particularly vowels, and have irregular articulation errors. When resonance is affected, ataxic dysarthria usually results in assimilated hypernasality. The speech of ataxic dysarthric patients is often called "scanning" and "singsong" referring to the patient's prosodic impairments. Patients with ataxic dysarthria produce speech slowly, often prolonging intervals between and within words, and have excess and equal stress (See Table 6.6).

Table 6.6: Motor Speech Processes and Speech Pathologies in Ataxic Dysarthria

Motor Speech Process	Motor Speech Pathologies
Respiration	Altered Smooth Cycling of Respiration
Phonation	Harsh Voice Quality Monopitch Monoloudness
Articulation	Imprecise Consonants Irregular Articulatory Breakdown Prolonged Phonemes
Resonance	Assimilated Hypernasality
Prosody	Slow Rate of Speech Prolonged Intervals Excess and Equal Stress

The prosodic aspect of speech is the prime carrier of the emotion of an utterance.

Movement Dysarthrias

The movement dysarthrias are caused by damage to the extrapyramidal system which consists of the basal ganglia, the substantia nigra, and parts of the brainstem. The function of the extrapyramidal system is to control postural reflexes and to facilitate and integrate muscle movements. The movement dysarthrias involve unwanted and defective speech movements which can occur slowly or rapidly. While muscle tone and coordination may also be affected in the movement dysarthrias, the speech pathologies primarily result from movement defects, impairments, and irregularities. The movement neuromuscular communication disorders are hypokinetic and hyperkinetic dysarthrias.

Hypokinetic Dysarthria

Although any disease process or disorder affecting the extrapyramidal system can cause hypokinetic dysarthria, *Parkinson's disease* is the primary cause of it. In 1817, James Parkinson published, "Essay on the Shaking Palsy" (Parkinson, 1817) and the disease has since been referred to by his name. Parkinson's disease is a degenerative disorder of the nervous system caused by abnormally low concentrations of dopamine and other neurotransmitters. Most epidemiological studies show that Parkinson's disease is more frequent in persons in the latter decades of life, usually with an onset after age 50, and affecting approximately 2 of every 1,000 people (Tanner, 1976).

Respiration is usually not affected significantly in hypokinetic dysarthria. Monopitch and monoloudness are phonatory deficits and patients with hypokinetic dysarthria may have harsh or breathy voice qualities often with voice tremor. Patients with hypokinetic dysarthria distort consonants although nasal resonance distortions rarely occur. The prosodic impairments include reduced stress, inappropriate silences, variable rate of speech, and in Parkinson's disease, short rushes of speech, i.e., the *acceleration phenomenon*. Associated symptoms include tremor and the *on-off phenomenon* (akinesia paradoxica) which is the rapid spontaneous fluctuation of symptoms. Table 6.7 shows the salient speech pathologies in hypokinetic dysarthria.

Table 6.7: Motor Speech Processes and Speech Pathologies in Hypokinetic Dysarthria

Motor Speech Process	Motor Speech Pathologies
Respiration	Negligible Impairment
Phonation	Monopitch Monoloudness Harsh Voice Quality or Continuous Breathiness
Articulation	Imprecise Consonants
Resonance	Unaffected
Prosody	Reduced Stress Inappropriate Silences Variable Rate of Speech Short Rushes of Speech (Acceleration Phenomenon)

Hyperkinetic Dysarthria

Also a disorder of the extrapyramidal system, two types of hyperkinetic dysarthria are recognized: quick and slow. According to Duffy (2005), hyperkinetic dysarthria accounts for about 21.6% of all dysarthrias. The incidence and prevalence of hyperkinetic dysarthria are much higher if spasmodic dysphonia of neurologic origin and organic voice tremor are included: 26% of all dysarthrias. Hyperkinetic dysarthria may be caused by a variety of diseases and disorders and usually involves a reduction in neurotransmitters that inhibit neuromuscular involuntary movements.

The designation of quick and slow are relative and on a continuum. Both types of abnormal excessive involuntary movements affecting speech may be present in a particular patient. (In addition, technically hypokinetic dysarthria involving the effects of abnormal, excessive unwanted movements on speech production may also be considered a slow hyperkinesia). As Darley, Aronson, and Brown (1975) observed, these dysarthrias are better labeled "predominately" quick or slow (See Table 6.8).

Table 6.8: Primary Hyperkinesias

Predominantly Quick Hyperkinesias	Characteristics
Myoclonic Jerks (Myoclonus)	Sudden, Unsustained Muscle Contractions
Tics	Rapid, Unsustained, Nonrhythmic Muscle Contractions
Chorea	Irregular Rapid Muscular Contractions (Sustained or Unsustained)

Predominantly Slow Hyperkinesias	Characteristics
Athetosis	Slow Writhing Movements
Dystonia	Waxing and Waning of Speech Mechanism Postures
Dyskinesis	Quick or Slow and Regular or Irregular Unwanted Muscle Movements
Tremor	Series of Rhythmic, Purposeless Muscle Oscillations
Spasmodic Dysphonia (Neurologic Origin)	Voice Pathologies Due to Laryngospasms

Predominantly Quick Hyperkinetic Dysarthrias

Myoclonic jerks (myoclonus), *tics*, and *chorea* are major predominantly quick hyperkinesias resulting in abnormal excessive involuntary muscle movements. When these muscle movements affect respiration, phonation, articulation, resonance, or prosody, hyperkinetic dysarthria results.

Myoclonic jerks, unsustained sudden contractions of muscles large enough to move a body part, can randomly affect one or several muscles and occur on one or both sides of the body. They may also affect one muscle and systematically spread to others. Myoclonic jerks may happen infrequently or repeatedly. Seizures, strokes, infections, poisoning, and tumors may cause myoclonus.

Tics are nonrhythmic, rapid and unsustained muscle contractions. They may be neurologically-based or psychological in origin. "They tend to be associated with an irresistible urge to perform them and often can be voluntarily suppressed temporarily" (Duffy, 1995, p. 192). *Gilles de la Tourette's syndrome* is a major cause of tics affecting speech production. The onset of Tourette's syndrome is in early childhood with changes in the severity of the symptoms often occurring in adolescence. Symptoms of this genetic disorder include facial grimacing, vocal tics, grunts, barking, sniffing, and explosive vocalizations. *Coprolalia*, uncontrolled, repetitive swearing behavior, is a common although not universal symptom of Tourette's syndrome.

> Hiccups are examples of myoclonic jerks of the respiratory process because of spasms of the diaphragm.

Chorea, sometimes called "St. Vitus' dance disease" is a movement disorder caused by a variety of etiological factors including degenerative diseases, infections, metabolic, and toxins. Its symptoms include random, purposeless movements of a body part often occurring rapidly. When these involuntary movements involve the motor speech processes, significant deviations in speech production occur including articulatory distortions, voice quality changes, hypernasality, and pitch and loudness irregularities.

Other movement disorders that may result in quick hyperkinetic dysarthrias include *ballism*, involuntary large thrashing and jerky movements, *spasms*, sudden involuntary contraction of a muscle or groups of muscles, and muscle *fasciculations*, small involuntary muscle contractions. When these movements affect the motor speech processes, they can cause speech pathologies ranging in severity from mild voice and articulation impairments to reduced intelligibility.

Predominantly Slow Hyperkinetic Dysarthrias

While some authorities do not make the quick-slow distinction regarding hyperkinetic dysarthria, the slow hyperkinesias of *athetosis* and *dystonia* have salient features that clearly distinguish them as slow rather than fast unwanted involuntary muscular movements. They are characterized by slowly developing muscle contractions which are sustained for at least one second, and in some instance, several minutes. In addition, muscle tone waxes and wanes which produces postural distortions (Darley, Aronson, and Brown, 1975). *Dyskinesia* may be considered a fast or slow hyperkinesia with an abnormally variable rate and rhythm of movement (Duffy, 2005). *Tremor*, a series of rhythmic, purposeless, muscle oscillations, and *spasmodic dysphonia of neurologic origin* can also be considered predominantly slow hyperkinetic dysarthrias.

Athetosis is characterized by repetitive slow, twisting, writhing movements primarily of the limbs but also of the face and head. Athetosis is caused by cerebral palsy but it can also result from strokes and other diseases and disorders affecting the extrapyramidal system. Most of the research on the speech pathologies associated with athetosis has been conducted on children and adults with athetoid cerebral palsy. The research suggests athetosis interferes with normal respiration, phonation, articulation, and prosody for speech production purposes. Primarily, athetosis disrupts breathing cycles, voice quality, pitch and loudness, articulatory precision, and rate of speech.

Dystonia is considered the slowest of the movement disorders (Darley, Aronson, and Brown, 1975). Also resulting from damage to the extrapyramidal system, it is characterized by sustained contractions causing twisting and writhing movements. When dystonia affects the respiratory, phonatory, and articulatory muscles, speech production is impaired. According to Duffy (1995, p. 207), the primary speech pathologies associated with dystonia include voice quality impairments, audible inspiration, voice tremor, hypernasality, speech sound distortions, inappropriate silences, and "excessive-inefficient-variable" patterns of stress.

Dyskinesia is a general category of neuromuscular impairments which can be quick or slow and regular and irregular. Long-term antipsychotic and other medication regimens cause *tardive dyskinesia*. Abnormal involuntary muscle movements may affect just the tongue, face, and jaw or be more generalized. Articulation and prosody are primarily affected in *orofacial dyskinesias*.

Tremor is an unwanted, relatively rhythmic muscle oscillation causing a shaking movement of one or more body parts. More than 20 types of tremor have been identified and most are normal occurrences in healthy people (National Institute of Neurological Disorders and Stroke, 2007). Both normal and abnormal tremors may be *postural* (static) and occur when a body part is maintained against gravity, *resting*, when a body part is at rest, and *terminal*, occurring toward the end of a movement. *Essential tremor* is the most common type usually affecting the hands but also the head, larynx, and tongue (National Institute of Neurological Disorders and Stroke, 2007). Mild tremors which do not substantially move body parts do not cause speech pathologies. However, moderate and severe tremors may impair normal speech and voice production.

According to Duffy (2005), spasmodic dysphonia of neurologic origin has distinguishing characteristics of hyperkinetic dysarthria. The primary perceptual features involve phonation-respiration (impaired voice quality, voice tremor, strained phonation), resonance (occasional intermittent hypernasality and nasal emission), and articulation-prosody (inappropriate silences, short phrasing). The speech pathologies involved in spasmodic dysphonia of neurologic origin are primarily due to laryngospasms.

> The first symptom of a progressive neurogenic communication disorder may be abnormal voice.

Mixed and Multiple Dysarthrias

Mixed and multiple dysarthrias result from damage to more than one neurological system and include more than one of the previously discussed pure dysarthrias. Mixed and multiple dysarthrias also occur when a dysarthria evolves over time from one diagnostic category to another. According to Duffy (2005), mixed dysarthrias are common and occur at a rate higher than for any single type: 29.1% of all dysarthrias. Mixed and multiple dysarthrias are caused by multiple strokes, degenerative conditions, traumas, tumors, inflammatory processes, and other diseases and disorders that can affect multiple neurological systems. Two major causes of mixed and multiple dysarthrias are *amyotrophic lateral sclerosis* (ALS) and *multiple sclerosis* (MS).

Amyotrophic lateral sclerosis is commonly referred to as "Lou Gehrig's" disease because the famous baseball player contracted it.

Amyotrophic lateral sclerosis is a neurodegenerative disease affecting both upper and lower motor neurons of the brain and spinal cord and causing spastic-flaccid dysarthria. Currently, there is no known cause of the disease, although a small percentage of ALS cases appear to be hereditary. Currently, there are few treatments for ALS, however, gene therapy is showing promise as an effective treatment.

"It is important to recognize that dysarthria in ALS may not be perceived as mixed at all points during the disease. It may present either flaccid or spastic dysarthria; when mixed, one type may predominate" (Duffy, 1995, p. 244). As such, the dysarthric symptoms in amyotrophic lateral sclerosis may present as primarily pure flaccid or spastic and progress into multiple neurological system impairments. The speech pathologies of ALS can impair all of the motor speech process of respiration, phonation, articulation, resonance, and prosody. Consequently, patients in the late states of amyotrophic lateral sclerosis have significantly reduced intelligibility and many are rendered anarthric.

Multiple sclerosis results in mixed and multiple dysarthria of the ataxic-spastic type. Multiple sclerosis is a demyelinating (damage to the protective myelin sheath surrounding nerves) usually striking people between 20 and 40 years of age. The cause of MS is unknown although current research suggests it may be an autoimmune disorder. The neurological symptoms of multiple sclerosis include nystagmus (involuntary rhythmic shaking of the eyes), tremor, gait disturbances, and sensory impairments. Although MS may affect cognitive functions such as memory and perception, it is primarily a motor disorder. Approximately 50% of patients with multiple sclerosis have dysarthria.

The dysarthria symptoms seen in multiple sclerosis are variable and can range from mild articulatory movement disruptions and voice quality impairments to significantly reduced intelligibility. Multiple sclerosis can impair pitch and loudness control, articulation precision, resonance, and prosody. "Severity of dysarthria in MS is positively related to severity of neurologic involvement. Most speech deviations become more prominent as additional motor systems become involved" (Darley, Aronson, and Brown, 1975, p. 243).

Other causes of mixed and multiple dysarthrias include *Wilson's disease, Friedreich's ataxia, progressive supranuclear palsy, Shy-Drager syndrome,* and *olivopontocerebellar atrophy* (Duffy, 2005, 1995). Wilson's disease is a genetic metabolic disorder affecting the processing of copper. Friedreich's ataxia is an inherited progressive ataxia. Shy-Drager syndrome is a progressive disorder of the autonomic and central nervous system. Olivopontocerebellar atrophy as the term suggests, is degeneration of neurons in the cerebellum, pons, and inferior olivary nuclei in the brainstem. The above diseases may affect multiple motor systems and consequently result in mixed and multiple dysarthrias.

Efficacy of Dysarthria Treatment

In the past 50 years, much research has been conducted on dysarthria treatments. Many studies have been completed on the dysarthrias in general and speech pathologies associated with specific diseases such as Parkinson's disease, multiple sclerosis, cerebral palsy, and others. However, few studies on the efficacy of dysarthria treatment use control groups (Joffe and Reilly, 2003). While there has been no comprehensive study analyzing general efficacy of all dysarthria treatments, or a meta-analysis of previous studies, most studies show that motor speech therapies improve speech production. This is not surprising because dysarthria therapies are based on physical therapy treatment principles and there is a large body of evidence that they improve muscle strength, tone, range-of-motion, etc. Those improvements can be extrapolated to dysarthria treatments albeit with qualifications that many speech muscles cannot be directly accessed physically.

> Early initiation of dysarthria treatment is particularly important in many degenerative neurogenic communication disorders to slow speech deterioration and the decline of intelligibility.

Of the research conducted on the efficacy of dysarthria treatments, many concentrate on children. "There is limited evidence that treatment programmes developed specifically for children with motor speech disorders (either dyspraxia or dysarthria) are any more efficient than other 'traditional' articulation or phonological programmes" (Joffe and Reilly, 2003, p. 247). However, Robertson (2001) shows that orofacial motor speech exercises are beneficial especially when accompanied by follow-up home-based drills and exercises. Below are therapeutic activities that can be supported by family members of a stroke patient but also is applicable to dysarthrias of other etiologies (Tanner, 2007, pp. 189-191).

> **Slowing the Rate of Speech:** In most activities, the faster a person does something the less precise he or she is at doing it; hence the old adage, "Haste makes waste." The faster you try to wash dishes, mow the lawn, or paint a house, the less care and precision goes into it. The same principle holds true for speaking. The faster a person talks, the less precisely each individual sound is made. When speaking becomes faster than about 600 words a minute, most people become unintelligible. For many stroke survivors, reducing the rate of speech helps them adjust for muscle weakness or paralysis of the speech system. Slowing the rate of speech helps the stroke survivor relearn how to produce each individual sound clearly and precisely. As the patient progresses in his or her rehabilitation program, he or she can begin to talk progressively faster once again.
>
> **Exaggerating Individual Sounds:** Speech can often be improved significantly by teaching the patient to exaggerate each individual sound. Although the patient may find it difficult to get into the habit of exaggerating each sound while talking, after a while it becomes second nature, and the more the patient exaggerates the sounds, the better speech becomes.

Clearly Producing the Final Sounds of Words: In normal speech, there is a tendency to produce the first sound of a word more clearly than the sounds that occur in the middle or at the end. When the stroke survivor with dysarthria is encouraged to produce the final sounds of a word as clearly as he or she does the other ones, speech improves, sometimes dramatically.

Opening the Mouth More Widely: A singer opens his or her mouth more widely to allow the voice to radiate out more effectively. For a stroke survivor with dysarthria, it is also sometimes helpful to learn to open the mouth wider when speaking. This allows the patient to produced sounds more clearly and reduces the tendency to muffle speech. Opening the mouth more widely also helps the patient to remember to slow his or her speech and to exaggerate each sound.

Speaking Louder: Speech has to be of sufficient loudness to be understood. No matter how clearly or precisely the sounds are made, speech will fall on "deaf ears" if it is not made loud enough. Sometimes just having the stroke survivor sit or stand with an erect posture helps increase loudness.

Working on Specific Sounds: For many dysarthric patients, the sounds made by having the tongue reach the top of the mouth are the most difficult to make. Particularly troublesome are those sounds produced at the top and at the front of the mouth such as *t, th,* and *d.* As a result, the speech-language clinician may want the patient to do specific exercises to strengthen and improve the movement of the tongue. Most of the time, these exercises are speech drills, but sometimes nonspeech activities are used, such as trying to touch the nose with the tongue or sticking the tongue out as far as possible. However, it is usually best to give the patient speech exercises rather than nonspeech ones because speech exercises transfer more naturally to speaking situations.

Setting Standards: Sometimes just having the patient try harder to clearly produce speech will result in significant improvement. One way of doing this is to set up a number system that reflects the patient's increased efforts. A scale of 1 to 10 works best. On this 1 to 10 continuum, the number 5 represents normal, easy, effortless way people usually make their sounds. The number 1 is speech that cannot be understood and is produced in a slurred, distorted manner. The number 10 represents per. . . fect . . . ly . . . ar . . . tic . . . u . . . la . . . ted . . . sp . . . ee . . . ch in which every sound is made with the absolute amount of precision that is humanly possible. Setting the goal of an 8 or 9 standard, and praising the stroke survivor for trying to reach it, results in higher levels of speech precision, as well as providing a way of measuring and rewarding improvement.

Principles of Evaluation and Treatment for the Dysarthrias

Principle 1: An initial dysarthria screening and quick assessment should be conducted rather than a comprehensive diagnostic test.

As has been emphasized throughout this text, the practice of comprehensively assessing neurogenic communication disorders immediately post onset and using the diagnostic information as a basis for treatment, is clinically inappropriate. With the dysarthrias, in particular, the initial symptoms are likely to change significantly over time. Even patients with *stable dysarthria*, whose neuromuscular impairments have remained relatively consistent, will have some change in the disorder due to the effects of therapies, changes in medication, and as a result of spontaneous recovery. Consequently, a brief initial dysarthria screening test should be administered during the initial bedside evaluation, and therapeutic evaluation should be ongoing and integral to each session. A modified Likert scale continuum (1 = clearly abnormal or nonfunctional to 5= clearly normal or functional) to assess the patient's motor speech production abilities can be used to test for dysarthria. Screening tests can give the clinician adequate information to begin diagnostic therapy (Tanner and Culbertson, 1999).

Principle 2: Operant condition techniques are optimal treatment methods for the dysarthrias.

Operant conditioning, using rewards for gradual improvement of motor speech behaviors, is the best behavioral management approach for the dysarthrias. The treatment involves immediate rewarding of desired behaviors, or close approximations to them, cues and prompts, and the use of schedules of reinforcement to improve neuromuscular abilities.

Principle 3: The fundamental treatment objectives for the dysarthrias are dependent on their specific classification: paralytic, coordination, and movement dysarthrias.

While all dysarthria treatments involve comprehensive improvement of neuromuscular speech production abilities, the fundamental objectives are based on whether the disorder is primarily a result of muscular paralysis, disruptions in speech coordination, or a movement disorder. The primary treatments address specific paralytic, coordination, and movement disruptions affecting the patient's five basic motor speech process: respiration, phonation, articulation, resonance, and prosody.

> "Communication-oriented treatment may improve communication even when speech itself does not improve. It includes a variety of modifications ranging from altering the number of listeners, the amount of noise, speaker-listener distance, and eye contact to informing new listeners about the speech problem, its cause, and the speaker's preferred method of communicating" (Duffy, 1995, p. 378).

Principle 4: The treatment of predominantly paralytic dysarthrias (flaccid, spastic, and unilateral upper motor neuron) requires management of range of motion, muscle tone, and strength of muscular movements.

Range of motion of a body structure concerns muscle flexion and extension. Muscle spasticity, in particular, reduces range of motion, and can impair virtually all of the motor speech processes. Exercises to gradually increase range of motion are important to the treatment of spastic dysarthria. Therapies for predominantly paralytic dysarthrias also address the tone (tension or resistance to movement) of speech production muscles. Goals include improvements in the ability of muscles to respond to stretching. Muscle strengthening exercises are also primary goals of predominantly paralytic dysarthria treatments. While the above can be addressed independently, drills and exercises can be effectively combined to improve range of motion, muscle tone, and strength of muscular movements.

Principle 5: The treatment of the coordination neurogenic communication disorder, ataxic dysarthria, primarily addresses the direction, timing, force, and rhythm of motor speech production movements.

The primary treatment objective for ataxic dysarthria is to improve coordination of speech production muscle movements. As such, the goal is to improve the direction, timing, force, and rhythm of speech production muscle movements. This is accomplished by the patient slowing his or her rate of speech and making conscious purposeful speech acts accompanied by careful self-monitoring. Gradually, as the patient improves speech coordination, he or she can increase rate of speech with more precise muscle direction, timing, force, and rhythm.

> Rate of speech is dependent on the length and number of pauses, and the duration of the syllable.

Principle 6: The treatment of predominantly movement neurogenic communication disorders (hypokinetic and hyperkinetic dysarthrias) emphasizes reducing or eliminating unwanted movements and integrating appropriate muscle motions into speech acts.

The movement dysarthrias result from neurotransmitters abnormalities. Because therapeutic activities cannot substantially increase or decrease neurochemicals, the principle treatment goal is for the patient consciously to compensate for abnormal neuromuscular actions. This requires that he or she increase the division of attention from content to manner of speech production with an emphasis on decreasing speech distortions and reduction or elimination of unwanted movements. Speech drills provided frequently and in short sessions emphasizing conscious compensation and self-monitoring are essential to the treatment of all dysarthrias but particularly the movement neurogenic communication disorders.

Principle 7: Dysarthria treatments can and should be integrated into treatments for concomitantly occurring neurogenic communication disorders.

Treatment goals, objectives, and procedures discussed in the aphasic language encoding disorders (See Chapter 3) and verbal apraxia (See Chapter 5) can be integrated into dysarthria therapies. Any therapeutic exercise requiring the patient to speak can also include secondary goals emphasizing range of motion, muscle tone and strength, coordination, and the reduction or elimination of unwanted movements.

Principle 8: Therapeutic management of dysarthria requires establishing baselines, increasing physiologic support, conscious compensation, and extensive speech practice (Duffy, 2005).

Baselines are necessary for establishing goals and measuring changes. The patient should consciously compensate for motor speech production impairments, engage in extensive drills, and improvement quantified based on baseline measurements. Figure 6.1 provides principles of treatment.

| An initial dysarthria screening and quick assessment should be conducted rather than a comprehensive diagnostic test. |
| Operant condition techniques are optimal treatment methods for the dysarthrias. |
| The fundamental treatment objectives for the dysarthrias are dependent on their specific classification: paralytic, coordination, and movement dysarthrias. |
| The treatment of predominantly paralytic dysarthrias (flaccid, spastic, and unilateral upper motor neuron) requires management of range of motion, muscle tone, and strength of muscular movements. |
| The treatment of the coordination neurogenic communication disorder, ataxic dysarthria, primarily addresses the direction, timing, force, and rhythm of motor speech production movements. |
| The treatment of predominantly movement neurogenic communication disorders (hypokinetic and hyperkinetic dysarthrias) emphasizes reducing or eliminating unwanted movements and integrating appropriate muscle motions into speech acts. |
| Dysarthria treatments can and should be integrated into treatments for concomitantly occurring neurogenic communication disorders. |
| Therapeutic management of dysarthria requires establishing baselines, increasing physiologic support, conscious compensation, and extensive speech practice. |

Figure 6.1: Principles of dysarthria treatment.

Chapter Summary

The dysarthrias result from damage to the central or peripheral nervous system and can affect respiration, phonation, articulation, resonance, and prosody. They can be classified as paralytic, coordination, and movement neurogenic communication disorders with therapeutic goals and procedures based on this classification system. The paralytic dysarthrias require management of range of motion, muscle tone, and strength of muscular movements during speech production.

Ataxic dysarthria, a coordination dysfunction, addresses the direction, timing, force, and rhythm of motor speech production movements. Treatment of the movement dysarthrias emphasizes reducing or eliminating unwanted movements and integrating appropriate muscle motions into speech acts. The goals and procedures to treat the dysarthrias can be incorporated into other therapies for neurogenic communication disorders such as aphasia and motor speech programming disorders.

Study and Discussion Questions

1. Summarize the motor speech production laws and theories for each of the motor speech processes.

2. What are the paralytic dysarthrias? Describe the therapeutic goals and procedures to treat them.

3. What is the coordination dysarthria? Describe the therapeutic goals and procedures to treat it.

4. What are the movement dysarthrias? Describe the therapeutic goals and procedures to treat them.

5. What are the mixed and multiple dysarthrias? Describe the therapeutic goals and procedures to treat them.

6. Provide examples of how dysarthria goals and procedures can be incorporated into other therapies for neurogenic communication disorders.

7. Describe therapeutic activities that can be supported by family members of a dysarthric patient.

8. List and discuss the principles of dysarthria evaluation and treatment.

Reference

Darley, F., Aronson, A., and Brown, J. (1975). *Motor speech disorders.* Philadelphia: W. B. Saunders.

Duffy, J.R. and Folger, W.N. (1986, November). Dysarthria in unilateral central nervous system lesions. Paper presented at the annual convention of the American Speech-Language-Hearing Association. Detroit.

Duffy, J. R. (1995). *Motor speech disorders: Substrates, differential diagnosis, and management.* St. Louis: Mosby.

Duffy, J.R. (2005). *Motor speech disorders: Substrates, differential diagnosis, and management* (2nd ed.). St. Louis: Mosby.

Haynes, W. O. and Pindzola, R. H. (2004). *Diagnosis and evaluation in speech pathology* (6th ed.). Boston: Pearson Allyn & Bacon.

Joffe, B. and Reilly, S. (2003). The evidence base for the evaluation and management of motor speech disorders in children. In S. Reilly, J. Douglas, and J. Oates (Eds). *Evidence based practice in speech pathology.* London: Whurr Publishers.

Landau, W.M. (1988). Ataxic hemiparesis: Special delux stroke or standard brand? *Neurology* 38:1799-1801.

National Institute of Neurological Disorders and Stroke (2007). NINDS Tremor Information Page. Retrieved June 21, 2007 from the World Wide Web: http://www.ninds.nih.gov/disorders/tremor/tremor.htm

Parkinson, J. (1817). *An essay on the shaking palsy.* London: Sherwood, Neely, and Jones.

Robertson, S. (2001). The efficacy of oro-facial and articulation exercises in dysarthria following stroke. *Int J Lang Commun Disorders,* 36, Suppl:292-7.

Tanner, D. (1976). Spectrographic, pausimetric, and intelligibility measures in Parkinson's disease. *Doctoral Dissertation*, Michigan State University, East Lansing, Michigan.

Tanner, D. (2007). *The family guide to surviving stroke and communication disorders (2ⁿᵈ ed.)*. Boston: Jones and Bartlett.

Tanner, D. and Culbertson, W. (1999). *Quick assessment for Dysarthria*. Oceanside, CA.: Academic Communication Associates.

Zemlin, W. (1998). *Speech and Hearing Science: Anatomy and Physiology* (4th ed.). Boston: Pearson Allyn & Bacon.

Chapter Seven: Neurogenic Communication Disorders and Traumatic Brain Injury

> "Be faithful in small things because it
> is in them that your strength lies."
>
> Mother Teresa

Chapter Preview: This chapter examines the major neurogenic communication disorders caused by traumatic brain injury. There is a discussion of traumatic brain injury as a special category of neurogenic communication disorders and the effects of reduced or disordered consciousness on patients with aphasia, apraxia of speech, and the dysarthrias. The motion and forces associated with traumatic brain injury are described and the potential effects on the TBI survivor. Mental executive functions, orientation, and memory are discussed as they pertain the traumatic brain injuries. Issues related to posttraumatic psychosis and pediatric traumatic brain injury are discussed. Principle of evaluation and treatment of communication disorders associated with traumatic brain injury are also provided.

Traumatic Brain Injury as a Special Category of Neurogenic Communication Disorders

The symptoms of neurogenic communication disorders associated with traumatic brain injury (TBI) are often substantially different from what is seen in so-called "classic" aphasia, apraxia of speech, and the dysarthrias. Traumatic brain injuries often, but not always, reduce or impair the patient's *consciousness*; his or her awareness of self and the environment. Whether the major speech and language centers of the brain and the tracts leading to and from them are damaged, and the effects of the TBI on the patient's consciousness, can greatly affect the nature of the neurogenic communication disorders. There are three variations of neurogenic communication disorders associated with traumatic brain injury.

First, patients with focalized traumatic brain and nervous system damage affecting the major speech and language centers of the brain, and the tracts leading to and from them, can present with classic aphasia, apraxia of speech, and the dysarthrias. They have the types and symptoms of neurogenic communication disorders discussed in previous chapters of this book. Second, sometimes patients suffer traumatic brain injuries not affecting the major speech and language centers, and the tracts leading to and from them, but have reduced or impaired consciousness affecting mental executive function, orientation, and memory. Although they have communication disorders related to reduced or impaired consciousness, they do not have classic aphasia, apraxia of speech, and the dysarthrias. Third, many patients have traumatic brain injuries affecting the major speech and language centers of the brain, and the tracts leading to and from them, and also suffer from reduced or impaired consciousness. Consequently, the aphasia, apraxia of speech, and the dysarthrias are compounded and complicated by the reduced or impaired consciousness and are discussed in greater detail below.

The Traumatically Brain-Injured Person

According to the National Institute on Deafness and Other Communication Disorders (2007), approximately 500,000 Americans are hospitalized each year from traumatic brain injuries. About 10 percent of traumatic brain injured survivors have mild to moderate cognitive and communication disorders that interfere with independent living, and another 200,000 have severe impairments that may require institutionalization.

The incidence and prevalence of persons surviving traumatic brain injury has increased in recent years due to medical advances. This decrease in TBI related mortality is partially due to improved rapid emergency transportation services. According to Ghajar (2000), much of the improved success rates in treating traumatic brain injuries is due to maintaining oxygenated blood supply through a swollen brain. According to Douglas (2004), the care for a person with a traumatic brain injury can be upwards of $1.8 million. Ylvisaker, Szekeres, and Feeney (2001) note that direct medical costs associated with acute hospitalization and rehabilitation for TBI patients are $48.3 billion per year. About half of all traumatic brain injuries are the result of transportation injuries (Centers for Disease Control, 1997). Accidental falls, assaults, sports injuries, and war-related traumas also are frequent causes of traumatic brain injuries.

Many studies have examined the characteristics of persons who suffer traumatic brain injuries. Males, especially young ones, are at least twice as likely to suffer traumatic brain injuries than females. Males tend to be employed high-risk jobs such as the military, construction, and farming, and they engage in more risk-taking behaviors. The age group with the highest risk for traumatic brain injury is fifteen to twenty-four years of age (Kraus and Sorenson, 1994). Low socioeconomic status, being unmarried, poor social skills, low education levels, learning disabilities, and a history of psychological maladjustment are also positively correlated with the likelihood of suffering a traumatic brain injury.

> The *shaken child syndrome*, a cause of pediatric traumatic brain injury, occurs when an adult violently shakes a child as punishment or to stop him or her from crying.

All studies show that traumatic brain injuries are positively associated with high blood alcohol levels and drug abuse. Most patients with accident-related traumatic brain injuries have detectible blood alcohol levels at the accident scene and many are legally intoxicated. In addition, there is a high recidivism rate for people who suffer traumatic brain injuries. One of the main predictors that a person will suffer a TBI is a history of one; apparently patients who suffer traumatic brain injuries continue to engage in risky behaviors. Based on the factors associated with traumatic brain injury, the following is a profile of the typical TBI patient (Tanner, 2007, p. 94):

> A young single male with poor education and academic skills, working in a job where the risk of accidental injury is great, earning below average income, who engages in risk-taking behaviors while using alcohol or recreational drugs, and who has previously been admitted to a hospital for a traumatic head and neck injury.

> Not only is alcohol abuse positively associated with traumatic brain injury, alcoholism interferes with rehabilitation and the alcoholic has poor prognosis for optimal recovery.

Motion and Forces of Traumatic Brain Injuries

Externally induced tearing, shearing, and temporal-spatial pressure changes within the brain cause traumatic brain injuries. Traumatic head injuries can be categorized into *open-penetrating* and *closed* types. The nature and extent of the brain injury is dependent on the intensity of the motion and forces involved, site of impact, direction and rotation of the brain tissue, and/or the trajectory of the projectile or projectiles though the brain.

An open-penetrating head injury is one resulting from a projectile (missile) entering the brain or an opening of the cranium into the atmosphere due to an impact. Projectiles in open-penetrating traumatic brain injuries include shrapnel, bullets, nails, pebbles, and other solid objects. (A rapid pressure release from a blank gunshot and other sources can also enter and damage the brain). There is destruction of brain tissue at the site of the impact and further damage as the projectile travels through the brain. Open-penetrating head injuries are seen in war, industrial and farming accidents, drive-by shootings, and other violent acts. In events involving strong head impacts, sometimes the forces are so great that brain matter exudes from the cranium.

A blunt force impact causes the second type of traumatic brain injury and does not involve opening of the cranium into the atmosphere. Closed head injuries can also be caused by forceful shaking such as occurs in the *shaken child syndrome*. Automobile accidents, falls, and sport traumas are common causes of closed head injuries. As with open-penetrating traumatic brain injuries, the severity of the brain damage is also dependent on the location and intensity of the impact. Often in blunt force traumas, there is *diffuse axonal injury* involving a shearing of axons during rotational acceleration of the brain (Gillis and Pierce, 1996).

Ylvisaker, Szekeres, and Feeney (2001) summarize the primary and secondary impact damage caused by traumatic brain injury. With regard to primary damage from traumatic brain injury of the open-penetrating type, there are high and low velocity impacts. *High velocity impacts* involve the projectile entering the brain causing destruction of tissue around the projectile path. *Low velocity impacts* involve fracture of the skull with debris entering the brain and possible substantial destruction of tissue at the site of impact.

According to Ylvisaker, Szekeres, and Feeney (2001), in closed head injuries, there is *acceleration/deceleration* of the brain as a moving object hits a movable head, a moving head hits a stationary object, or the head is shaken violently. The brain damage is caused by movement of the brain within the skull. In a *non-acceleration* closed head injury, a moving object hits a fixed head causing an *impression trauma* with localized brain damage. *Ellipsoidal deformation* injuries involve a slow-moving object with a large surface area deforming the skull causing brain tissue to move outward from the center with damage to central structures. In closed head injuries, the brain may move linearly or angularly. *Linear velocity damage* is caused by the brain moving along a linear path. In *angular acceleration* brain damage, the brain rotates at an angle causing lacerations, abrasions, and shearing actions with diffuse axonal injury, hemorrhage, and cranial nerve trauma.

Ylvisaker, Szekeres, and Feeney (2001) list *hemorrhage, cerebral edema, intracranial pressure, hypoxic-ischemic damage,* and *seizure* as pathologic secondary events of traumatic brain injury and which contribute to the impairments. Hemorrhagic secondary brain damage can include extracerebral and intracerebral bleeding. Extracerebral hemorrhaging is bleeding into the meninges and intracerebral hemorrhaging is a bleed into brain tissue. Cerebral edema is common around the primary site of injury and is the accumulation of fluid between the brain and the skull. Cerebral edema contributes to increased intracranial pressure (ICP). Increased intracranial pressure, as the label suggests, is an increase of pressure within the skull due to the accumulation of blood and other fluids and which can interfere with blood circulation in the brain. Hypoxic-ischemic damage is reduced oxygenation to the brain associated with severe diffuse axonal injury. Seizures may be early or late onset and can complicate recovery. According to Ylvisaker, Szekeres, and Feeney (2001), two or more late-onset seizures constitute epilepsy.

High velocity impacts damage the brain at the site of the impact, which is called the *coup* injury, while damage opposite the initial point of impact is called the *contra coup* injury. Contra coup brain injuries are a result of recoil of the brain inside the skull and is a consequence of Newton's Third Law: *For every action, there is an equal and opposite reaction.* "The brain's large mass gives it considerable momentum. When the skull stops moving, the brain runs into it. Depending on how suddenly the skull slows down, this second, contrecoup blow to the brain can cause as much or more injury as the initial blow. Animals with less massive brains rarely suffer this type of injury" (Young and Geller, 2007, p. 232).

Reduced or Impaired Consciousness as a
Primary Feature of Traumatic Brain Injury

Much has been written about impaired mental executive functioning, behavioral problems, disorientation, memory loss, and reduced or impaired levels of awareness associated with traumatic brain injury. These factors can influence, sometimes dramatically, the patient's overall neurogenic communication disorders symptoms. However, impaired mental executive functioning, behavioral problems, disorientation, memory loss, and reduced or impaired levels of awareness associated with traumatic brain injury, and the influence they have on neurogenic communication disorders, have one factor in common: the patient's *consciousness*. As a result, it is necessary generally to discuss human consciousness and its role in thought and behavior before exploring the specific cognitive, psychological, and behavioral disabilities associated with traumatic brain injury.

Cognitive Neuroscience and Human Consciousness

Consciousness is simply defined as a person's awareness of self and the environment. However, the notion of human consciousness is integral virtually to all religions and philosophies. No other concept is more relevant about the nature of human existence, more important to understanding human thought, emotion, and behavior, than is consciousness. On a fundamental level, consciousness is simply an organism's level of *thoughtful arousal*, a product of the *sensorium*, a hypothetical part of the brain for the intellect, and the *reticular activating system,* which regulates arousal and wakefulness. And yet the implications of this self-awareness and responsiveness to the environment transcend the totality of a person's cognitive, emotional, and behavioral being. The origin of human consciousness is a hotly debated topic with theories ranging from a supernatural imposition to consciousness as a property of matter. Language plays an important role in the nature and manifestation of human consciousness.

All living organisms have degrees of consciousness with differing levels of awareness of self and the environment. Worms, birds, dogs, dolphins, and apes have unique levels of awareness of self and their surroundings. Humans have a high, if not the highest, level of awareness allowing them actively to integrate knowledge of the past and present with realistic appraisal of the future. This high level of consciousness permits, if not requires, humans purposefully to act on an ever-changing environment. Traumatic brain injury can disrupt, and sometimes eliminate, this self-awareness and purposeful interaction with the environment. Reduced or impaired consciousness arising from traumatic brain injury can affect the patient's mental executive functioning causing a myriad of behavioral problems, and lie at the core of his or her disorientation and amnesias. In the worst case scenario, traumatic brain injury can render a patient *comatose* and lacking of consciousness.

Coma, Persistent Vegetative States, Stupor, Delirium, and Clouding of Consciousness

A patient in a *coma* is unconscious and unable to respond to internal or environmental stimuli. A patient in a *persistent vegetative state* has lost his or her cognitive abilities and awareness of surroundings, but retains vegetative brain functions such as breathing, sleep patterns, and circulation. He or she may have spontaneous movements, the eyes may open in response to external stimuli, and have occasional grimacing, laughing, or crying (National Institute of Neurological Disorders and Stroke, 2007).

Other terms for reduced or impaired consciousness are less well-defined. A patient in a *stupor* has reduced or impaired consciousness requiring continued stimulation to show arousal and attention to the environment. A patient who is *delirious* has reduced or disordered consciousness accompanied by agitation. The clinical label for the least level of reduced or impaired consciousness is *clouding of consciousness*. A patient whose consciousness is clouded has mild levels of disorientation and confusion that fluctuate over time.

> While rare, there are several documented cases of patients awakening from lengthy comas with near-normal or normal cognitive functions. The film "Awakenings" is an account of a group of patients who regain awareness from a coma-like state.

Loss of Consciousness and Posttraumatic Amnesia as Indicators of Severity of Traumatic Brain Injury

Lucas (1998) reports that the time it takes for the patient to regain consciousness is predictive of the severity of the traumatic brain injury. If the patient is unconscious for fewer than thirty minutes, he or she has suffered a mild traumatic brain injury. On the other hand, if the length of unconsciousness exceeds thirty minutes, the survivor has suffered a moderate to severe brain injury.

Posttraumatic amnesia (PTA) is also an indicator of the severity of traumatic brain injury. Technically, posttraumatic amnesia is impairment of the ability to learn new information following a traumatic brain injury. As a predictor of severity of traumatic brain injury, posttraumatic amnesia is usually the length of time from unconsciousness to the patient's first recall of events following the injury. Lucas (1998) reports that when the length of PTA is less than 1 hour, the patient has a mild brain injury. One to 24 hours of post traumatic amnesia indicates the patient has moderate brain injuries, and patients with PTA longer than 24 hours to one week have severe brain injuries. In addition, very mild brain injuries are associated with PTA of less than five minutes and very severe ones are associated with PTA of 1-5 weeks. Lucas (1998) observes that the length of posttraumatic amnesia is a better predictor of severity of head injury than is length of unconsciousness. As a practical matter, however, traumatic brain injured persons are not good sources about the length of time they were unconscious or the duration of their posttraumatic amnesia.

The Glasgow Coma Scale and the Rancho Los Amigos Scale of Cognitive-Behavioral Functioning

The *Glasgow Coma Scale* (Teasdale and Gennet, 1974) is the most widely used neurological scale to assess consciousness and is also predictive of recovery. It assesses three categories of patient behavior: eye opening, verbalization, and motor responses.

In the category of *eye opening response*, a patient who has spontaneous eye opening with normal blinking receives 4 points. One who opens eyes to verbal commands, speech, or shouting, receives 3 points. The patient who opens his or her eyes to pain (not applied to the face) receives 2 points and 1 point is given for no eye-opening.

With regard to *verbal responses*, a patient who is oriented receives 5 points and one who is confused but answers questions receives 4 points. Inappropriate verbal responses that are intelligible receives 3 points while unintelligible speech is given 2 points. One point is given for no verbal responses.

Motor responses include 6 points for obeying movement commands, 5 points for purposeful movement to pain, and 4 points for withdrawal from pain. Abnormal (spastic) flexion responses (decorticate posture) receives 3 points, and the patient in decerebrate posture, with rigid extensor responses, receives 2 points. One point is give for no motor responses.

The total number of points are summed across each category: Total score = E+V+M. Patients with a score of 3-8 are in various levels of coma. The moderate range of impaired consciousness is 9-12 points and mild impairment is 13-15 points.

Another widely used rating scale for cognitive and behavioral functioning for traumatic brain injury is the *Rancho Los Amigos Scale* (Hagen, 1981). The assessment instrument does not require participation from the patient. "The scale is sometimes a frame of reference for characterizing phases of recovery" (Davis, 2007, p. 278). The eight levels include (See *Rancho Los Amigos Scale* for completed description of behavior, memory, and learning for each level):

I.   No Response: Patient unresponsive to all stimuli.
II. Generalized Response: Inconsistent, nonpurposeful, delayed, and/or gross responses.
III. Localized Response: May follow simple commands; responses specific but inconsistent.

IV. Confused-Agitated: Hyperactive responses, confusion, disorientation, uncooperative.

V. Confused-Inappropriate, Non-Agitated: Responses nonpurposeful, random; distractible.

VI. Confused-Appropriate: Some awareness of self, environment, and goal-directed behavior.

VII. Automatic-Appropriate: Basic orientation but lack of insight into condition.

VIII. Purposeful-Appropriate: Alert, oriented, good memory; poor stress tolerance.

The *Rancho Los Amigos Scale* is helpful for family members in understanding the stages of recovery from traumatic brain injury.

Traumatic Brain Injury, Impaired Mental Executive Functioning, and Metacognition

Many patients who suffer traumatic brain injury display behavior problems ranging from reduced inhibition and aggressiveness to indifference and *flat affect*, the lack of normal emotion. For some patients, these are chronic behavioral problems and for others, they are temporary and necessary stages of recovery from traumatic brain injury. These behavioral problems can be divided into *hyperfunctional* and *hypofunctional* behavior problems (See Table 7.1). Common types of behavior problems seen in some traumatic brain injured persons include making inappropriate sexual advances, aggressiveness, acting too friendly to strangers, impulsiveness, apathy, reduced spontaneity, and lack of interest in people, activities, and things that were once interesting to the patient.

Table 7.1: Hyperfunctional and Hypofunctional Behavior Patterns in Traumatic Brain Injury.

Hyperfunctional Behavior Patterns	Hypofunctional Behavior Patterns
Hypersexuality	Hyposexuality
Aggressiveness	Apathy
Mood Swings	Flat Affect
Impulsiveness	Reduced spontaneity
Increased socialness	Decreased socialness
Euphoria	Depression
Hyperattentive	Hypoattentive
Restlessness	Psychomotor retardation

Authorities on traumatic brain injury classify many of these behavior problems under the category of *impaired mental executive functioning*. The notion of mental executive functioning is drawn from business and likens a person's directing of attention, planning and initiation of behavior, and monitoring of his or her actions, to the function of a company's chief executive officer in running a company. A more encompassing term for mental executive function is *metacognition*, the process of "thinking about thinking" (Flavell, 1979). Problems with mental executive functioning and metacognition are associated with damage to the frontal and temporal lobes of the brain and in *frontal lobe syndrome* in particular. Frontal lobe syndrome is a collection of behavior problems following severe, diffuse bilateral damage to the frontal lobes; it is also called *apathetic-akinetic-abulic* syndrome.

Metacognition is necessary for optimal learning. It involves assessing the realistic nature of situations, acting appropriately, influencing the environment, and monitoring the success or failure of such actions. Metacognition, at a basic level, is necessary for traumatic brain injured persons to appropriately direct attention, realistically assess situations, resolve conflicts, monitor behaviors, and to profit from experience.

> Care must be taken when evaluating
> disorientation in TBI patients with aphasia.
> Verbal statements made by patients regarding
> time, place, person, and/or situation/
> predicament may be made with verbal
> paraphasias (association errors) suggesting
> that they are disoriented when, in fact, they
> are oriented but producing naming errors.

Traumatic Brain Injury, Disorientation, and Memory Loss

Many patients who suffer significant traumatic brain injury are confused and classified as disoriented to *time, place, person,* and/or *situation/predicament*. Patients who are disoriented to only one aspect of life are said to be "disoriented times one," patients disoriented to two aspects are "disoriented times two," and so forth. Rarely are patients with significant traumatic brain injuries only disoriented to either time, place, person, or situation/predicament. Most patients have general disorientation that transcends all aspects of their lives.

Many patients with significant traumatic brain injury are disoriented to time especially early post-onset. They are confused about time events and the passage of time. A patient disoriented to time may be confused about the year, season, month, or time-of-day. He or she may also believe that an hour has gone by, when in fact, only ten minutes have transpired. Disorientation to place may be manifest by the patient being confused about his or her room or the fact that he or she is in a hospital. Some patients are mixed-up about the city, state, or country in which they reside. While all types of disorientation can be unsettling for family members, the patient disoriented to person can be particularly distressing. A patient disoriented to person may believe his wife is his mother or that a current husband is actually a previous one. A traumatic brain-injured person who believes he or she is in the hospital for routine medical tests, when in fact, he or she is confined to a rehabilitation unit for a serious brain injury is confused about situation and predicament. Patients who are disoriented to situation/predicament often engage in denial of disability: *anosognosia*.

Some authorities on traumatic brain injury separate problems patients have with memory loss from the disorientation they may experience. However, memory loss and disorientation are integrally related; there is a strong relationship between memory and orientation. Simply stated, if a patient could remember accurately aspects of his or her life related to time, place, person, and/or situation/predicament, he or she would be basically oriented. This is not to say that all disorientation is a product of memory problems, only that they are fundamentally related. Ylvisaker, Szekeres, and Feeney (2001) report that memory deficits are among the most commonly reported problems in traumatic brain injury. They note that the memory problems experienced by TBI patients are related to hippocampus or frontal lobe damage.

Retrograde and Anterograde Amnesia

The time of the event causing a traumatic brain injury is the dividing line between two types of amnesia: retrograde and anterograde. *Retrograde amnesia* is general or specific loss of memory for events that occurred before the traumatic brain injury. The time period for lost memory can be one or two days or as long as decades. The patient with retrograde amnesia may have complete loss of memory or only blackouts for specific events. While all memory loss in traumatic brain injury is primarily due to damaged neurological tissue, psychological defense mechanisms and coping skills such as repression and denial also play a role.

Two popular films are excellent examples of retrograde and anterograde amnesias. *The Bourne Identity* is a film about a spy who suffers retrograde amnesia. *Memento* is about a person who cannot lay down new memories.

Anterograde amnesia is the impaired ability to acquire new memories. In traumatic brain injury, there are three components of information processing and memory that may breakdown: *attention, storage,* and *recall.* Breakdown at any level of memory can cause the inability to acquire new information, learn, and profit from therapeutic experiences. The initial and fundamental aspects of storing new information is dependent on the patient's ability to attend to self and the environment.

Attention

Attention is an important requisite to acquiring all learning and profiting from experience. For patients sufficiently to attend to self and the environment, they must have a basic state of *arousal*, the general state of readiness to process sensory input (Gillis, 1996). In traumatic brain injury, deficits at the attention level of memory can impede memory functions. Traumatic brain injured patients can be minimally impaired with regard to attending such as occurs with clouding of consciousness or they can be comatose and completely unaware of self and surrounding. The quantity and quality of information that is eventually stored and recalled is dependent on the patient's ability to attend to general and specific sensory information. Fundamental to an individual's ability to attend to self and environmental stimuli is the ability to separate the *figure* from the *ground.*

The concept of *figure-ground* involves an individual's ability to separate important salient aspects of the incoming stimuli from background or ambient information; it is sometimes compared to *signal-noise* concepts of information processing. In the auditory mode, the traumatic brain injured patient may have impairments with auditory perception. Although there is nothing wrong with the patient's hearing mechanism, he or she will be impaired or unable to separate important salient information from background noise. This can affect the patient's speech perception. In the visual mode, although there is nothing wrong with the patient's eyes, figure-ground deficits may impair his or her ability to attend visually to people, track their movements, and to read. Figure-ground problems can also occur with other sensory input, but deficits in the auditory and visual modes can significantly affect communication, learning, and the ability to profit from therapeutic exercises. Patients with traumatic brain injuries who cannot attend to important salient information can have memory functions impeded. Because incoming information is not made conscious or it is distorted, normal storage of new information does not occur.

> The common practice of leaving the television on in the hospital room may actually impair the TBI patient's ability to attend to important and salient information especially for those individuals with figure-ground deficits.

Storage

Storage of information occurs in the short and long term. *Short-term memory* is also called "working memory" and occurs for as long as the person rehearses what is to be remembered. Neurologically, short-term memory involves continuation of neural impulses. To test for short-term memory deficits, patients repeat digits forward and backward and recalls similar and dissimilar objects (Aronson, 2000). Icons are used to test visual short-term memory. Auditory short-term memory occurs for as long as the person rehearses the stimuli. Auditory short-term memory is seven plus or minus two digits controlled for speed of stimuli presentation. Controlling the speed of presentation of stimuli is important because of a phenomenon known as *chunking*, remembering a series of related units when said rapidly.

While short-term memory is the result of continuation of neural impulses, long-term memory is the result of changes in brain chemistry. The information is available for recall without rehearsal. Psychologically, the individual facilitates long-term memory making the stimuli personally relevant; he or she associates the new stimuli with previously stored information. Long-term memory can be *incidental* and *purposeful*. Incidental long-term storage of information occurs when there is no purposeful association by the individual. Long-term memory is purposeful when done by extensive rehearsal or by the use of *mnemonic devices*, the association new with previously stored and easily remembered information.

Recognition and Recall

The final components of normal memory are recognition and recall. Once information is attended to and stored, recognition and recall completes the memory process. However, it is unlikely that all information attended to and stored is available for recognition and recall because of psychological and organic factors. An important question about information processing and memory involves the subconscious mind: Is all information that is attended to and stored available for recognition and recall? This question addresses the psychological defense mechanism of *repression,* the blocking from conscious awareness memories, motivations, and information.

Repression is at the core of many defense mechanisms and coping styles. Repression blocks retrieval of disturbing and anxiety-provoking memories. Although these disturbing and anxiety-provoking experiences are attended to and stored, they are blocked from recall and conscious awareness. Synaptic dysfunctions, axon shearing and tearing, and neurochemical disruptions occurring in traumatic brain injury also interfere with the normal recall process. Recognition of stored information is easier than recall because the former supplies cues to the correct response while the latter requires all-inclusive retrieval of the information. In patients with traumatic brain injury, high scores in recognition and low scores in recall suggest unimpaired receptive vocabulary and deficient expressive abilities.

Traumatic Brain Injury and Psychosis

The data on the incidence of posttraumatic psychosis are highly variable (Smeltzer, Nasrallah, and Miller, 1994). As many as 20% of traumatic brain injured persons can be considered psychotic and upwards of 50% show signs and symptoms of the break with reality. The problems knowing the incidence and prevalence of posttraumatic psychosis are related to the definition of psychosis, accuracy of testing patients with communication disorders, and understanding some language disorders and the perception of reality.

Psychosis, a thought disorder, is a break with reality often accompanied by *hallucinations* and *delusions* and interfering with the individual's ability to test reality and function socially. A hallucination is a false or distorted interpretation of sensory information and can be visual, auditory, tactile-kinesthetic-proprioceptive, gustatory, and olfactory. A delusion is a fixed false belief rigidly held in proof to the contrary. Often in psychotic disorders, hallucinations and delusions occur concurrently. In traumatic brain injured persons, hallucinations and delusions may be a result of the nature, type, and site of brain lesions and/or psychogenic in nature. Psychologically, hallucinations and delusions may involve *projection*, the external attribution of one's own intolerable wishes, thoughts, motivations, and feelings. The most common hallucinations occurring in posttraumatic psychosis are visual and auditory.

Visual hallucinations involve the patient misinterpreting or have false images. He or she sees people and things that do not exist. Auditory hallucinations involve hearing nonexistent voices and environmental sounds. Visual and auditory hallucinations may be associated with several perceptual disorders resulting from traumatic brain injury and also concomitant symptoms of posttraumatic psychosis. In addition, paranoid, grandeur, and other delusional states may be a direct result of the traumatic brain injury or a concomitant symptom of posttraumatic psychosis.

> A mnemonic device for remembering the cranial nerves is "On old Olympus towering tops a Finn and German vended a hop. (Olfactory, Optic, Oculomotor, Trochlear, Trigeminal, Abducent, Facial, Auditory, Glossopharyngeal, Vagus, Accessory, Hypoglossal)

Traumatic brain injured persons with aphasia can be misdiagnosed as suffering from psychosis because of expressive language impairments, specifically verbal paraphasia (association errors). As reported in Chapters 2 and 3, a verbal paraphasia has a semantic relationship to the desired word, e.g., red for blue, top for bottom, dog for cat. A traumatic brain injured patient with a propensity to produce verbal paraphasias may say the incorrect word when naming or describing events. The patient may incorrectly describe an event using verbal paraphasias and lead the listener to conclude that what he or she is reporting is a delusion or hallucination and suffering from psychosis. However, in some cases, the patient may be reporting a real event but do so inaccurately because of his or her aphasia. In one such case, a patient reported being placed in a car and driven to a nearby fire station. In fact, the patient was describing a real event where he was transported to in his wheelchair to a glass-enclosed fire hose by the nursing station as a reward for good behavior. "Lane simply reported this event using aphasic paraphasias: *car* for *wheelchair*, *drove* for *wheeled*, and *fire station* for *fire hose*" (Tanner, 2006, p. 181).

Communication Disorders and Traumatic Brain Injury

As noted previously, communication abilities in persons with traumatic brain injury may be disrupted in three ways. As shown in Table 7.2, there are three primary variations of neurogenic communication disorders associated with traumatic brain injury.

Table 7.2: Three Variations of Neurogenic Communication Disorders Associated with Traumatic Brain Injury.

Focalized Traumatic Brain Injury Affecting the Major Speech and Language Centers/Tracts	Traumatic Brain Injury Not Affecting the Major Speech and Language Centers/Tracts	Diffuse Brain Injury Also Affecting the Major Speech and Language Centers/Tracts
Classic Aphasia Classic Apraxia of Speech Classic Dysarthria	Impaired or Disrupted Consciousness Affecting Mental Executive Functions, Orientation, and Memory	Aphasia, Apraxia of Speech, and the Dysarthrias Compounded and Complicated by Reduced or Impaired Consciousness

First, the patient may have only focalized damage to the major speech and language centers of the brain and the tracts leading to and from them. In these rare cases, the brain damage suffered by the patient is similar to the damage caused by a single focalized stroke. Consequently, patients display classic symptoms of the "big three" stroke-related neurogenic communication disorders: aphasia, apraxia of speech, and/or the dysarthrias. With regard to aphasia, these patients either have predominantly expressive or receptive language disturbances, more or less, cutting across all modalities of communication. They may display the seven types of wordfinding seen in classic aphasia: *mutism, literal phonemic approximations, verbal semantic associations, delay, description, generalization,* and *tip-of-the-tongue* behaviors (See Chapter 3). Other language disorders involving expressive and receptive phonology, syntax, and grammar are typical of what is seen in stroke-survivors with aphasia. In these patients, the language disorders are not affected by reduced or impaired consciousness and their communication disorders are typical of stroke patients with aphasia.

Patients with classic motor speech disorders have the complication errors, struggle, and other motor speech programming errors seen in many stroke-survivors with verbal apraxia. However, patients with reduced or impaired consciousness may display speech symptoms of ideational apraxia (See Chapter 5). The dysarthric symptoms occurring in focalized lesions depend on the site of lesion or lesions caused by the traumatic brain injury however, they are not complicated by reduced or impaired consciousness.

Second, the traumatic brain injury may spare the major speech and language centers of the brain and the tracts leading to and from them. The motor speech processes of respiration, phonation, articulation, resonance, and prosody may be programmed and executed normally and the fabric of language unimpaired by the traumatic brain injury. However, these patients display the impaired speech and language characterized by impaired or disrupted consciousness. The patient may have impaired or reduced awareness, problems testing reality, retrograde and anterograde amnesia, and disorientation. The diagnostic label given to patients with significant traumatic brain injury not affecting the major speech and language centers of the brain is the *language of confusion.* Table 7.3 shows the cognitive and behavioral disorders typically seen in patients with the language of confusion.

Table 7.3: Cognitive and Behavioral Disorders in the Language of Confusion

Function	Disorder	Description
Awareness	Coma, stupor, delirium, clouding of consciousness	Absent or reduced awareness of self and environment
Reality Testing	Posttraumatic psychosis	Break with one or more aspects of reality: Hallucinations and delusions
Memory	Retrograde and anterograde amnesia	Memory loss of events before and/or after the TBI, problems learning
Orientation	Disorientation to time, place, person, and/or situation (predicament)	Confusion about time events and/or the passage of time, people (including self), place, and the reason for hospitalization

Third, patients with significant traumatic brain injury often have diffuse brain damage affecting the major speech and language centers of the brain compounded and complicated by reduced or disordered consciousness. In effect, patients in this category show their awareness, reality testing, memory, and orientation impairments with defective language and/or motor speech production deficits. This is why many traumatic brain injured patients have atypical and sometimes bizarre communication disorders. While the most common linguistic impairment in closed head injury is anomia (Hartley and Levin, 1990), it is in the area of language pragmatics that patients with classic aphasia and head injury most contrast (Holland, 1982). Davis (2007) suggests three discourse and conversation targets in traumatic brain injured patients: theory of mind (ability to take the perspective of another for making inferences), thematic coherence, and conversational management. Specifically, patients display pragmatic deficits regarding controlling emotions, focusing attention, sustaining attention, memory, and executive initiation of conversations.

Traumatic brain injuries can damage the external, middle, and inner ear, and according to Northern and Downs (1991), meningitis can be a late complication of temporal bone fractures. Patients with traumatic brain injury should undergo some type of risk assessment screening to determine the possibility of damage to the hearing mechanism (Mackay, Chapman, and Morgan, 1997. Audiology testing is an important part of the management of traumatic brain injury to determine the status of the hearing mechanism and to rule out hearing loss and deafness as a variable in speech and language and neuropsychological testing. If a hearing loss is detected, then appropriate treatment should be part of the overall rehabilitation program.

> Bleeding in the middle ear or disruption of the ossicular chain can create a maximal 60-dB conductive hearing loss (Northern and Downs, 1991).

Pediatric Traumatic Brain Injury

"Closed-head trauma in children is a major public health problem. It is a leading cause of death among youth and results in substantial neurobehavioral morbidity for survivors" (Yeates, 2000, p. 92). While children with traumatic brain injury share commonalities with adults, they pose unique challenges and opportunities for rehabilitation specialists. Damage to an immature brain results in different TBI symptoms than what occurs in a mature one. Conventional thought among rehabilitation specialists is that because children's brains are more pliable and uncommitted, they have much better prognoses than their adult counterparts. While there is some truth to this observation, children may be more vulnerable than adults in certain critical areas of functioning (Ylvisaker, 1998). Children have not fully developed a learning style and most return to school involving formal instruction. Additionally, children are not as emotionally mature as adults and they are also more dependent on peer approval and acceptance. An important variable in pediatric traumatic brain injury is "when" during the development period the child suffers the injury.

In the United States, pediatric traumatic brain injury spans from birth to age 18 years. Children below the age of eight (approximately) who suffer traumatic brain injury will have communication disorders significantly influenced by the interruption of normal speech and language developmental milestones acquisition. Although there is great variability in the rate normal children develop communication abilities, by approximately age eight, most children will have acquired the fundamental aspects of speech and language (Tanner, Culbertson, and Secord, 1997; Tanner, Lamb, and Secord, 1997). Although semantic learning continues throughout life, the essential aspects of grammar, syntax, and the acquisition of speech sounds are essentially complete by approximately age eight. Consequently, the younger the child, the more likely the traumatic brain injury will interfere with the acquisition of normal communication developmental milestones. In addition, children suffering traumatic brain injuries affecting the major speech and language centers of the brain, and the tracts leading to and from them, will be more communicatively compromised than those with brain damage not involving them. Besides disrupting the acquisition of communication developmental milestones, pediatric traumatic brain injuries interfere with attention, episodic memory, behavioral organization, and learning new information (Davis, 2007).

> The number-one cause of traumatic brain injury in children is high-speed automobile accidents (Snow and Hooper, 1994).

Efficacy of Traumatic Brain Injury Treatment

A common statement made about the traumatic brain injured patient is "Rehabilitation begins at the scene of the accident." To insure that all that can be done for the patient is done for him or her, an early start is beneficial and the more intensive the treatment, the better the outcomes.

Many health care professionals may be involved in the evaluation and treatment of traumatic brain injured patients. For patients with only focalized damage to the major speech and language centers of the brain and the tracts leading to and from them, the speech-language pathology service may be the primarily professionals involved in rehabilitation. Because these patients display classic aphasia and motor speech disorders, they are evaluated and treated similarly to stroke-survivors.

For patient with communication disorders directly or indirectly affected by reduced or impaired consciousness, the *rehabilitation team* provides a cohesive and integrated evaluation and treatment program. Although the members of the rehabilitation team will vary depending on the nature of patients' head injury, core members include specialists from physiatry (rehabilitation medicine), nursing, psychology, rehabilitation counseling, social work, audiology, food and nutrition sciences, and occupational, physical, and speech services.

Some hospitals and rehabilitation centers provide formal or informal *coma stimulation therapy* for patients with reduced or impaired consciousness. Coma stimulation therapy is the multisensory stimulation to improve the patient's awareness, orientation, memory, and learning. In coma stimulation therapy, various odors and fragrances to the nose, tastes on the tongue, temperature contrasts to the skin, and speech and nonspeech stimulation to the ears are provided to patients in various degrees of coma (Baker, 2007; Gillis, 1996). Other activities included in some coma stimulation therapies include exposure to bright colors, reading to the patient, providing information about current events, contrasting hot and cold stimulation to the skin, and range-of-motion exercises. The benefits of coma stimulation have not been conclusively demonstrated, especially concerning deep comas, and currently, the therapy is considered experimental. A drawback of the coma treatment is that it may reinforce denial and create false hopes for the patient's family and friends.

Reality orientation is a procedure involving the entire rehabilitation team and the family of the head injured patient. In reality orientation therapy, the patient is regularly and consistently given relevant information about the date and time, reasons for the patient being in the facility, his or her location, and other important information regarding time, place, person, and situation (predicament). One goal of reality orientation therapy is to reduce the duration of the patient's posttraumatic amnesia. De Guise, Leblanc, Feyz, Thomas, and Gosselin (2005) found clinically relevant but not statistically significant shorter posttraumatic amnesia in traumatic brain injured subjects receiving reality orientation. Reality orientation therapy requires regular communication among the rehabilitation team so that the information provided to the patient is consistent, meaningful, and relevant to his or her goal and objectives.

Ylvisaker and Szekeres (1994) emphasize the importance of building a positive self-concept for the traumatic brain injured patient. It is important that rehabilitation tasks be consistent with the patient's premorbid personality and interests. They note that rehabilitation success requires appropriately adjusted expectations and improves the self-concept of the patient. Ylvisaker and Feeney (1998) propose that self-awareness, setting of reasonable goals, appropriate planning and organization, and effective monitoring of performance be addressed in the treatment of executive function disorders.

> Frequently, family members of the patient report that memory impairments and behavior changes are two persistent residual impairments of significant traumatic brain injury.

Principles of Evaluation and Treatment of Communication Disorders Resulting from Traumatic Brain Injury

Principle 1: An initial traumatic brain injury screening and quick assessment should be conducted rather than a comprehensive diagnostic test.

Ongoing evaluation of communication disorders in traumatic brain injured patients is essential to adapt treatments to their changing levels of arousal and consciousness. With the exception of patients in deep comas, most traumatic brain injured patients will have significant changes in their speech and language, attention, orientation, memory, and behavior.

Principle 2: Ongoing evaluation of the patient should separate classic aphasia, apraxia of speech, and dysarthria from general attention, orientation, memory, and behavior disorders resulting from the traumatic brain injury.

To the extent possible, disorders of language and motor speech should be identified and separate goals and objectives of treatment be established to address them. Making this clinical distinction is challenging especially for patients whose reduced and disordered consciousness significantly compounds and complicates the language and motor speech production disorders. Treatment goals and procedures for symptoms of classic aphasia are provided in Chapter 3, for motor speech programming disorders in Chapter 5, and for the dysarthrias in Chapter 6.

Principle 3: Coma stimulation is an experimental therapy with little justification for patients in deep comas, but possibly beneficial for patients in less significant states of reduced or impaired consciousness.

No conclusive data shows the benefit of coma stimulation for patients in deep comas. However, patients with less significant reductions or impairments of consciousness may benefit from it. Coma stimulation should always include ongoing assessment of the patient's ability to profit from the experience.

Principle 4: Speech and language rehabilitation goals and objectives should be incorporated into reality orientation procedures.

For patients with impaired language and motor speech production disorders, reality orientation procedures should incorporate aphasia and motor speech programming and execution drills and exercises. Language and motor speech production goals and objectives should be integrated into reality orientation procedures while addressing issues related to time, place, person, and situation (predicament).

Principle 5: The treatment of communication disorders associated with traumatic brain injury should actively involve the patient's family members, other health care professionals, and the utilization of speech-language pathology assistants.

Most rehabilitation programs rely on the team approach to dealing with traumatic brain injured patients. Consequently, health care professionals will communicate regularly about the goals, objectives, and treatment procedures for TBI patients. Inclusion of the patient's family members in the ongoing evaluation and treatment of communication disorders related to traumatic brain injury is necessary and warranted because family members typically spend much time with the patient. Knowledgeable and involved family members can conduct routine coma stimulation drills and exercises and provide valuable assistance in reality orientation programs. In addition, because some treatment procedures for severely involved head injured patients require basic and simple drills and exercises, speech-language pathology assistants can provide cost-effective clinical services.

Principle 6: All therapeutic activities should directly or indirectly address realistic home or employment settings for the patient.

Inpatient therapeutic activities should be practical; they should deal with skills and functions necessary for the patient to return to employment and independent home living. Therapeutic activities should be related to the patient's vocation/profession, hobbies, and living arrangements.

Principle 7: The primary long-term rehabilitation goal in traumatic brain injured persons with reduced or disordered consciousness is to improve mental executive functioning (metacognition).

Primary to normal or functional metacognition is the patient's mental flexibility. Therapeutic activities should focus on planning, initiating action, monitoring behaviors, and evaluating outcomes.

Principle 8: Important factors to consider in determining the traumatic brain injured patient's discharge to home, and the required level of support and supervision, is his or her mental competence and safety risks to self and others.

The patient's legal mental competence concerning finances, employment, driving, and participation in legal proceeding are primary factors to evaluate by the rehabilitation team. In addition, a case-by-case determination must be made to decide whether the patient, upon discharge, is a danger to himself or herself and the necessary level of support and supervision. Figure 7. 1 provides principles of treatment for communication disorders associated with traumatic brain injury.

An initial traumatic brain injury screening and quick assessment should be conducted rather than a comprehensive diagnostic test.
Ongoing evaluation of the patient should separate classic aphasia, apraxia of speech, and dysarthria from general attention, orientation, memory, and behavior disorders resulting from the traumatic brain injury.
Coma stimulation is an experimental therapy with little justification for patients in deep comas, but possibly beneficial for patients in less significant states of reduced or impaired consciousness.
Speech and language rehabilitation goals and objectives should be incorporated into reality orientation procedures.
The treatment of communication disorders associated with traumatic brain injury should actively involve the patient's family members, other health care professionals, and the utilization of speech-language pathology assistants.
The primary long-term rehabilitation goal in traumatic brain injured persons with reduced or disordered consciousness is to improve mental executive functioning (metacognition).
Important factors to consider in determining the traumatic brain injured patient's discharge to home, and the required level of support and supervision, is his or her mental competence and safety risks to self and others.

Figure 7.1: Principles of treatment for communication disorders associated with traumatic brain injury.

Chapter Summary

The communication disorders associated with traumatic brain injury are a special category of neurogenic communication disorders. Some patients have traumatic brain injuries resulting in classic aphasia, apraxia of speech, and the dysarthrias. Other patients have the major speech and language centers of the brain, and the tracts leading to and from them, spared by the traumatic brain injury and have communication disorders primarily related to reduced and impaired consciousness. These patients may have behavioral problems, disorientation, memory loss, and reduced or impaired levels of awareness. Many TBI patients have aphasia, apraxia of speech, and the dysarthrias complicated and compounded by the reduced and impaired consciousness. Coma, persistent vegetative states, stupor, delirium, clouding of consciousness, and posttraumatic psychosis are also aspects of traumatic brain injury.

Study and Discussion Questions

1. Describe the "classic" neurogenic communication disorders and explain how they may result from traumatic brain injuries.

2. List and discuss the hyperfunction and hypofunctional behavior patterns in traumatic brain injury.

3. Describe the *Glasgow Coma Scale*.

4. Describe the *Rancho Los Amigos Scale*.

5. What are metacognition and mental executive functioning and how might be they breakdown in traumatic brain injured patients?

6. List and describe the components of memory and related them to traumatic brain injury.

7. What is posttraumatic psychosis?

8. Compare and contrast pediatric and adult traumatic brain injury.

9. Why should audiological screens be conducted on traumatic brain injured patients?

10. List and discuss the principles of treatment for communication disorders associated with traumatic brain injury.

References

Aronson, A.E. (2000). *Aronson's neurosciences pocket lectures: Speech, language, voice.* San Diego: Singular.

Baker, J. (2007). Explaining coma arousal therapy. *Coma Recovery Association.* Retrieved July 30, 2007 from the World Wide Web: http://www.comarecovery.org/comaarousal.shtm.

Centers for Disease Control (1997). Traumatic brain injury-Colorado, Missouri, Oklahoma, & Utah, 1990-1993. *MMWR, 46,* 8-11.

Davis, G.A. (2007). *Aphasiology: Disorders and clinical practice* (2nd ed.) Boston: Pearson, Allyn and Bacon.

De Guise, E. Leblanc, J., Feyz, M., Thomas, H., and Gosselin, N. (2005). Effect of an integrated reality orientation programme in acute care on post-traumatic amnesia in patients with traumatic brain injury. *Brain Injury,* Volume 19, Issue 4: 263 - 269.

Douglas, J. (2004). The evidence base for the cognitive-communicative disorders after traumatic brain injury in adults. In *Evidence based practice in speech pathology,* S. Reilly, J. Douglas, and J. Oates (Eds). London: Whurr Publishers.

Flavell, J. H. (1979). Metacognition and cognitive monitoring: A new area of cognitive-developmental inquiry. *American Psychologist,* 34, 906-911

Gillis, R., and Pierce, J. (1996). Mechanism of traumatic brain injury and the pathophysiologic consequences. In R. Gillis (Ed), *Traumatic brain injury rehabilitation for speech-language pathologists.* Boston: Butterworth-Heinemann.

Ghajar, J. (2000 September 9). Traumatic brain injury. *Lancet, 356*: 923-29.

Gillis, R. (1996). *Traumatic brain injury rehabilitation for speech-language pathologists.* Boston: Butterworth-Heinemann.

Hagen, C. (1981). Language disorders secondary to closed head injury: Diagnosis and treatment. *Topics in Language Disorders*, 1, 73-87.

Hartley, L. and Levin, H. (1990). Linguistic deficits after closed head injury: Current appraisal. *Aphasiology*, 4, 353-370.

Holland, A. (1982). When is aphasia aphasia? The problem of closed head injury. In R. L. Brookshire (Ed), *Clinical aphasiology conference proceedings* (pp. 345-390). Minneapolis, MN.

Kraus, J. and Sorenson, S. (1994). Epidemiology. In J. Silver, S. Yudofsky, and R. Hales (Eds) *Neuropsychiatry of traumatic brain injury.* Washington, DC: American Psychiatric Press.

Lucas, J.A. (1998). Traumatic brain injury. In P. Snyder and P.D. Nussbaum (Eds), *Clinical neuropsychology: A pocket handbook for assessment.* American Psychological Association: Author.

Mackay, L., Chapman, P., & Morgan, A. (1997). *Maximizing brain injury recovery: Integrating critical care and early rehabilitation.* Gaithersburg, MD: Aspen.

National Institute on Deafness and Other Communication Disorders (2007). Traumatic brain injury: cognitive and communication disorders. Retrieved June 28, 2007 from the World Wide Web: http://www.nidcd.nih.gov/health/voice/tbrain.htm.

National Institute of Neurological Disease and Stroke (2007). NINDS coma and persistent vegetative state information page. Retrieved July 6, 2007 from the World Wide Web: http://www.ninds.nih.gov/disorders/coma/coma.htmgf

Northern, J., & Downs, M. (1991). *Hearing in children* (4th ed.). Philadelphia: Lippincott Williams & Wilkins.

Smeltzer, D., Nasrallah, H., and Miller, S. (1994). Psychotic disorders. In J. Silver, S. Yudofsky, and R. Hales (Eds) *Neuropsychiatry of traumatic brain injury.* Washington, DC: American Psychiatric Press.

Snow, J. and Hooper, S. (1994). *Pediatric traumatic brain injury.* Thousand Oaks, CA: Sage

Tanner, D., Lamb, W., and Secord, W. (1997). *Cognitive, Linguistic and Social Communication Scales (CLASS)* (2nd ed.). Oceanside, CA: Academic Communication Associates.

Tanner, D., Culbertson, W., and Secord, W. (1997). *Developmental Articulation and Phonology Profile (DAPP).* Oceanside, CA: Academic Communication Associates.

Tanner, D. (2006). *Case studies in communication sciences and disorders.* Upper Saddle River, N.J.: Pearson Merrill Prentice Hall.

Tanner, D. (2007). *The medical-legal and forensic aspects of communication disorders, voice prints, and speaker profiling.* Tucson: Lawyers and Judges.

Teasdale, G. and Jennet, B. (1974). Assessment of coma and impaired consciousness: a practical scale, *Lancet* 2:81-84.

Yeates, K. (2000). Closed-head injury. In K. Yeates, M. Ris, and H. Taylor (Eds.), *Pediatric neuropsychology.* New York: Guilford Press.

Ylvisaker, M., & Szekeres, S. (1994). Communication disorders associated with closed head injuries. In R. Chapey (Ed.), *Language intervention strategies in adult aphasia* (3rd ed.). Baltimore: Williams & Wilkins.

Ylvisaker, M. and Feeney, T.(1998). *Collaborative brain injury intervention.* San Diego: Singular.

Ylvisaker, M., Szekeres, S.F., and Feeney, T. (2001). Communication disorders associated with traumatic brain injury. In *Language intervention strategies in aphasia and related neurogenic communication disorders* (4th ed.), R. Chapey, (Ed). Philadelphia: Lippincott Williams & Wilkins.

Young, H. and Geller, R. (2007). *Sears & Zemansky's college physics* (8th ed.). San Francisco: Pearson, Addison Wesley.

Part II

The Psychology of Neurogenic Communication Disorders

Chapter Eight: Psycho-Organic Determinants

"But it must be said from the outset
that a disease is never a mere loss or
excess–that there is always a reaction,
on the part of the affected organism
or individual, to restore, to replace, to
compensate for and to preserve its identity,
however strange the means may be."

Oliver Sacks, *The Man Who Mistook His Wife for a Hat*

Chapter Preview: This chapter examines the psycho-organic determinants associated with neurogenic communication disorders. Psychological generalities are made based on the type and location of brain damage and involving emotional lability, catastrophic reactions, perseveration, organic depression-anxiety disorder, anosognosia, homonymous hemianopsia and visual neglect, and euphoria. Also addressed are the behavioral and adjustment problems associated with Wernicke aphasia and traumatic brain injured patients.

Multiple Determinants of the Psychology of Neurogenic Communication Disorders

Currently, there are three determinants for the psychological impairments and adjustment challenges facing patients with neurogenic communication disorders: *psycho-organic, impaired defenses,* and *response to loss*. First, as discussed in this chapter, brain damage causing neurogenic communication disorders may directly affect the patient's psychological well-being. Injury to the brain can cause or be associated with psychological reactions including euphoria, psychosis, anxiety, depression, denial, and others. An otherwise psychologically healthy person who suffers brain damage can be significantly and negatively affected by these psycho-organic factors. Second, neurogenic communication disorders can be substantial psychological stressors and tax the patient's premorbid coping styles and psychological defenses. In the case of aphasia, verbal coping styles and psychological defenses can be impaired or eliminated because of the loss of language and leave the patient without habitual methods of adjusting to the disorders (See Chapter 9). Third, as reported in Chapter 10, most patients suffering significant neurogenic communication disorders experience loss of physical and mental abilities, valued objects, and are communicatively separated from loved ones. They can be expected to grieve over the unwanted changes associated with the neurogenic communication disorders and pass through predictable stages of grief. In many cases of neurogenic communication disorders, psycho-organic, impaired defenses, and the response to loss combine to affect the patient's psychology and adjustment to the disorders (See Figure 8.1). "For many individuals the psychological sequelae following a neurological injury are at least as debilitating as the actual physical symptoms" (Tetnowski, 2003, p. ix).

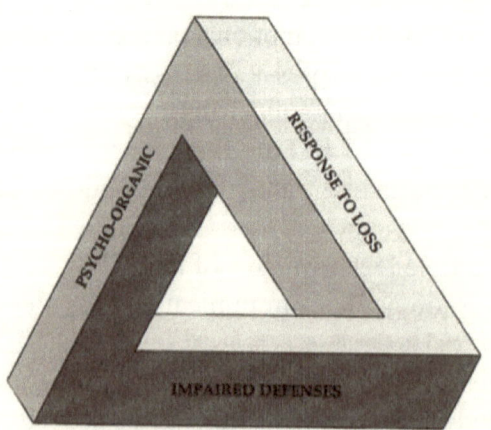

Figure 8.1: Three aspects of the psychology of neurogenic communication disorders

Psycho-Organic Determinants and the Localization Movement

The psycho-organic determinants to the psychology of neurogenic communication disorders are a direct result of brain injury. The role brain damage plays in the psychology of neurogenic communication disorders has been studied for decades and is closely tied to the localization movement discussed in Chapter 2. Today, a great deal of research is being conducted on the site of brain injury associated with or causing psychological reactions. The goal is to identify areas of the brain causing psychosis, aggression, denial, depression, euphoria, and many other psychological reactions. Strict localizationists believe that all significant psychological reactions can be traced to specific parts of the brain and that depression, anxiety, psychosis, and so forth, are directly caused by brain injury. Other localizationists, gestaltists, acknowledge that injury to parts of the brain are associated with many psychological reactions, but are not the absolute cause of them. A good example of the localization versus holistic view of the psychology of neurogenic communication disorders is clinical depression.

To strict localizationists, the clinical depression seen in patients with neurogenic communication disorders is a direct result of damage to specific parts of the brain. The brain damage causes a deficiency of certain neurochemical associated with a sense of well-being and results in depression often accompanied by anxiety. The treatment for this psycho-organic depression is the administration of antidepressants which corrects the neurochemical imbalance. Gestaltists, on the other hand, acknowledge the role brain damage plays in the onset of clinical depression in patients with neurogenic communication disorders, but also consider the role stress, loss and grief, and impaired defense mechanisms and coping styles play in clinical depression. Gestaltists believe that antidepressants should be combined with counseling, psychotherapy, life-style changes, and other social treatments for depression. Some authorities label the localization school of thought, the *medical model*, while the gestaltist philosophy is sometimes referred to as the *social model*. Currently, much research is being conducted into these issues with often controversial and inconclusive results.

> The term "psyche" is Greek in origin and refers to the human "mind" and "soul."

Brain Damage as a Predisposing Factor in the Psychology of Neurogenic Communication Disorders

When addressing the psycho-organic determinants in the psychology of neurogenic communication disorders, the *predisposing, precipitating,* and *perpetuating* factors associated with brain injury must be addressed to explain the adjustment challenges and psychological disorders experienced by some patients. Although brain damage may precipitate and perpetuate psychological disorders and maladjustment to neurogenic communication disorders, it is best viewed as a predisposing factor. A precipitating factor is an important or necessary condition to cause a psychological disorder or to set a maladaptive response into motion. A perpetuating factor causes the psychological reaction or disorder to be persistent or permanent. Predisposing factors, brain damage, incline a patient to a particular psychological condition, attitude, or behavior.

Because of brain damage, patients with neurogenic communication disorders can be predisposed to certain psychological reactions and disorders. A good example of the predisposing factor of temporal lobe damage is aggressive, violent, and impulsive behavior. Tardiff (1997) and others, have found that injury to the temporal lobes cause aggression and a propensity for violence. Temporal lobe epilepsy is associated with purposeless violence and has been used as a defense in legal cases (Tanner, 2007). Some legal authorities have proposed that violent offenders have inherited brain irregularities leading to a propensity for criminal behavior. As with most localization research, studies addressing aggressive, violent, and impulsive behavior often result in disparate and sometimes contradictory results. Frontal lobe damage has also been linked to aggressive, violent, impulsive, and other dissocial behaviors. However, it is well-documented that brain injury can predispose a person to certain dissocial behaviors. Importantly, it should be noted that while some individuals with temporal and frontal lobe damage become violent offenders, most do not. Consequently, psycho-organic determinants are best viewed as predisposing factors requiring precipitating, perpetuating, and other yet to be discovered phenomena to account for maladjustment and psychological disorders in neurogenic communication disorders.

Generalities About Brain Injury and Psychological Reactions

Certain generalities can be made about the nature, type, and location of brain injury and their predisposing effects for certain psychological reactions in patients with neurogenic communication disorders Tanner (2009), Tanner (2007), Williams, Evans, and Fleminger (2003), Carota, Rossetti, Karapanayiotides, and Bogousslavsky, (2001), Ylvisaker, Szekeres, and Feeney (2001), Tardiff, (1997), Gordon, et al. (1996), Tanner and Gerstenberger, (1996), Smeltzer, Nasrallah, and Miller (1994), Gainotti, (1989), Robinson, et al., (1988), Lipsey, et al., (1986), Robinson, (1986), Robinson, et al., (1985), Gordon, et al., (1985), Sackeim and Weber, (1982), Sackeim, et al, (1982), Robinson and Benson, (1981), Gasparini, et al., (1978), Black, (1975), Weinstein and Puig-Antich, (1974), Gainotti, (1972), Weinstein, et al., (1966), and others. It is important to note that many adjustment challenges and psychological disorders predisposed by brain injury are not substantially different from the kinds of reactions seen in psychologically disturbed people without brain damage (functional disorders).

Table 8.1: Type and Location of Brain Injury and Psychological Generalities

Type and Location Of Brain Injury	Psychological Generalities

Traumatic Brain Injury	Neuropsychological Deficits Not Typically Seen in Stroke Including:
	    -Posttraumatic Psychosis
	    -Amnesia and Disorientation
	    -Behavior Disorders
	Differences in Open and Closed Head Injury Symptoms Initially with Diverging Manifestations Overtime

Stroke	Long-Lasting Depression
Left-Hemisphere Damage	Anxiety Depression
Right-Hemisphere Damage	Indifference Apathy Cheerfulness Euphoria
Posterior Left-Hemisphere	Indifference Anosognosia Euphoria
Anterior Left-Hemisphere	Anxiety Depression
Wernicke's Area	Anosognosia Indifference Euphoria
Broca's Area	Short-Lived Emotional Outbursts Anxiety Depression

As Table 8.1 shows, traumatic brain injury is associated with cognitive, memory, learning, and orientation deficits not typically seen in strokes. Initially, open and closed head injuries tend to present with similar psychological symptoms, but as time passes, they diverge in their symptomatology. Approximately 50% of people who have communication disorders resulting from stroke will experience long-lasting depression. Regardless of etiology, patients with left-hemisphere brain damage are predisposed to anxiety and depression while those suffering right-hemisphere injury are more likely to be indifferent, apathetic, cheerful, and even euphoric. When the brain injury is in the posterior part of the left hemisphere, patients are predisposed to indifference, anosognosia (lack of awareness or denial of disability), and euphoria. When the brain injury is to the anterior part of the left-hemisphere, as many as 70% of patients are likely to experience depression often with accompanying anxiety. Damage to Wernicke's area predisposes patients to anosognosia. Damage to Broca's area is associated with short-lived emotional outbursts, anxiety, and depression and smaller brain lesions generally result in more awareness of disability than larger ones, likely contributing to the patient's frustration, anxiety, and depression. Figure 8.2 shows the approximate location of certain psychological reactions in some patients with neurogenic communication disorders.

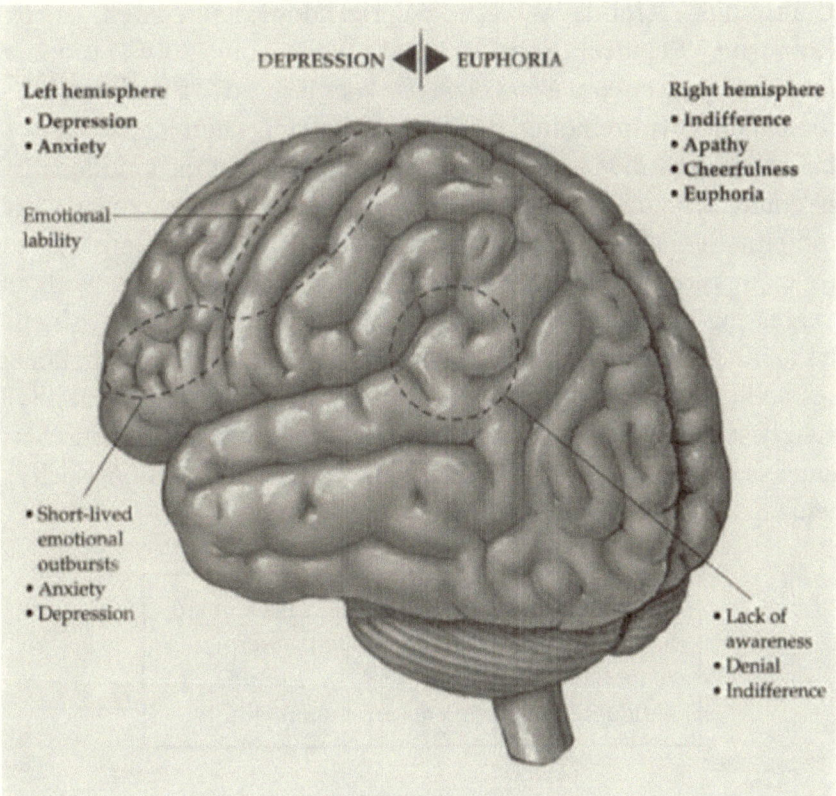

Figure 8.2: Approximate sites in the brain associated with psychological reactions in some patients with neurogenic communication disorders

Emotional Lability

Several terms are used to describe *emotional lability*, the involuntary exaggerated emotionality seen in some patients with neurogenic communication disorders: pseudobulbar emotional lability, inappropriate crying, pseudobulbar affect, pathological emotionality, uncontrolled emotional expression, and emotional incontinence. Bilateral brain damage causes emotional lability, and it occurs in several diseases and disorders including stroke, traumatic brain injury, Alzheimer's disease, and amyotrophic lateral sclerosis. In neurogenic communication disorders, emotional lability is often seen in spastic dysarthria (See Chapter 6) and bilateral damage to the motor strips of the brain and associated corticobulbar tracts.

Cummings, Arciniegas, Brooks, Herndon, Lauterbach, Pioro, Robinson, Scharre, Schiffer, and Weintraub (2006) propose *involuntary emotional expression disorder* be used as a unifying label for patients with emotional lability following neurological injury. Unfortunately, the label inaccurately suggests that the emotionality is completely involuntary when most patients can exercise some Inhibitory control. The label also indicates that emotions are limited to expression when patients can experience emotions without expressing them. The conventional label, emotional lability, should be retained because it accurately addresses the notion of emotional instability without unnecessarily limiting its parameters. "Lability" simply suggests "unstable" and "nonfixed," does not address etiology, and it is commonly used to describe other medical conditions such as wide blood pressure fluctuation.

> In a study done by Scoppetta, Di Gennaro, and Scoppetta (2005), a selective serotonin reuptake inhibitor (SSRI), a type of antidepressant, prevents emotional lability.

Although the research is unequivocal that brain damage predisposes patients to emotional lability, there is controversy concerning whether patients actually have true emotions associated with the acts of uncontrolled crying. Some authorities describe emotional lability as pathological emotionality without the authentic emotions linked to the stimuli that prompt the outbursts. Other authorities suggest that while involuntary emotional expressions occur in excess, most patients have normal underlying affect.

Regardless of the terms used to describe involuntary emotions occurring in neurological diseases and disorders, it should be noted that emotional lability is *exaggerated* and not *inappropriate* emotionality. Stimuli prompt the uncontrolled exaggerated involuntary emotional reactions and patients have lowered emotional thresholds for expression. Certainly, the emotions are excessive and usually involve crying because of the negativity associated with the patient's predicament. To propose that the crying behavior in these patients is "inappropriate" rather than "exaggerated" diminishes the patient's psychological response to his or her neurogenic communication disorders. In addition, assuming that all emotional reactions by the patient are pathological and inappropriate can create conditions where important quality of life issues for the patient are intellectualized and dismissed by health care professionals.

The triggers for emotional lability are similar to the stimuli causing emotional responses in normal persons. The patient's thoughts, certain situations, and highly charged words can set off bouts of emotional lability. Negative thoughts, particularly about the patient's predicament, can cause crying and many depressed patients are more likely to exhibit emotional lability. Excessive crying can alert health care professionals to a patient's underlying clinical depression. Situational triggers for emotional lability include visits by family and friends and frustrating therapeutic exercises. Gainotti (1989) suggests that emotional lability is a manifestation of a *catastrophic reaction*, a type of anxiety attack, in patients prone to crying (See below). In therapeutic activities and conversations with the emotionally labile patient, certain words can prompt crying. Highly charged and emotional terms such as "nursing home," "stroke," and names of loved ones can stimulate exaggerated emotionality in some patients.

In some patients, particularly those with severe and prolonged emotional lability, medication may be necessary to treat it successfully. Physicians may prescribe antidepressants or other medications to reduce or eliminate the patient's underlying negativity and anxiety. However, even in these patients, therapeutic intervention can precede or accompany pharmacological treatment. Duffy (2005) observes that emotional lability occurring during speech can have a significant negative effect on intelligibility. The "Three P" therapy for emotional lability, addressing the *predisposing, precipitating,* and *perpetuating* factors, can easily be incorporated into therapy for patients with communication disorders and reduce the frequency and duration of crying episodes.

While brain damage itself is the primary predisposing factor in emotional lability, other factors make a patient more susceptible to excessive crying. Negative sleeping habits, lack of exercise, poor diet, and stress can exacerbate emotional lability in many patients. To reduce the predisposing factors in emotional lability, attempts should be made to see that the patient gets plenty of sleep, exercises regularly, has a good diet, and efforts should be made to keep stress at a minimum. Additionally, there is a natural reduction in the predisposing factors for emotional lability because of spontaneous recovery (See Chapter 3) which occurs in most patients with neurogenic communication disorders.

The second aspect of the therapeutic management of emotional lability concerns the precipitants or triggers that set off bouts of exaggerated crying. As discussed above, thoughts, certain situations, and highly charged words can trigger excessive crying. Early post onset, attempts should be made to avoid as many situations and conversational triggers as possible. If possible, the patient should be counseled to redirect his or her thoughts to positive ones and away from negativity. As the patient regains emotional stability, he or she can gradually and systematically be exposed to the precipitating factors.

Perpetuating factors of emotional lability involve aspects of the behavior that cause the crying to continue excessively. Redirection of the patient's attention can reduce the length and severity of bouts of emotional lability. Patients can be instructed to direct their attention to pleasant thoughts and positive images during episodes of emotional lability to reduce the duration and severity of the episodes.

The *Three P Therapy* for emotional lability reduces or eliminates predisposing, precipitating, and perpetuating factors associated with emotional lability. It can be an effective treatment for patients with mild to moderate emotional lability. For patients with severe and prolonged emotional lability, it can be used in conjunction with medication management to help patients with neurogenic communication disorders regain emotional stability.

Catastrophic Reactions

According to Frank (1998), anxiety disorders include phobias, acute stress disorders, generalized anxiety disorders, post-traumatic stress syndrome, obsessive-compulsive disorders, and panic attacks. A *catastrophic reaction* is one manifestation of a panic attack occurring in some patients with neurogenic communication disorders. The catastrophic reaction usually occurs when the patient is confronted with too much stimuli and faced with the likelihood of failure. At the core of the catastrophic reaction is the patient's loss of a sense of mental and physical integrity and communicative impotence. A catastrophic reaction may occur during speech and language therapy when too much is required of the patient and communicative failure is likely. Research shows that catastrophic reactions are more likely to occur in patients with damage in and around Broca's area and resulting nonfluent speech output (Carota, Rossetti, Karapanayiotides, and Bogousslavsky, 2001). Post stroke depression and the occurrences of catastrophic reactions may be associated (Craig and Cummings, 1995). Depression and a propensity for catastrophic reactions may be related to the fact that anxiety is often a component in post stroke depression and that nonfluent aphasia is frustrating.

Jon Eisenson (1984) examined the catastrophic reaction in aphasic patients and considered it a *psychobiological breakdown*. The patient's panic is accompanied by physiological reactions such as increased blood pressure, muscular hypertension, sweating, and dry mouth. In extreme catastrophic reactions, a patient may strikeout physically and verbally, cry, and even lose consciousness. At the core of the physiological reactions in the catastrophic reaction is the *fight or flight response*. Physiologically, the patient prepares to flee or fight the perceived threat. Laraia (1998) notes that a panic attack occurs when the human alarm system is triggered. While excessive therapeutic stimuli may prompt a catastrophic reaction, too much visual clutter and ambient noise my also trigger one.

Prevention is the best treatment for catastrophic reactions. Unfortunately, it may take one or more occurrences of observable catastrophic reactions before the clinician is aware that a patient is prone to them. When the patient is experiencing a catastrophic reaction, the clinician should provide immediate reduction in the stimuli and provide an avenue for him or her to escape such as leaving the room or closing eyes and resting. The clinician can also provide soothing, comforting, and calming statements. Katz (2000) suggests a key parameter in treating the catastrophic reaction is addressing environmental factors. Relaxation training may also be helpful in patients with the communicative abilities to benefit from it.

Excessive intake of caffeine can trigger panic attacks.

Perseveration

Perseveration is the tendency for a person to inappropriately continue an act for a longer duration than is warranted by the significance of the stimulus that prompted it. *Echolalia,* a manifestation of recurrent perseveration (See below), is when a patient automatically repeats the sound, word, or phrase spoken by someone else. *Mitigated echolalia,* a normal process, is when a person repeats the last thing spoken by someone else when bidding for time to process information. Psychologically, echolalic responses occur in many patients to fill silences and to give the appearance of normalcy. Perseveration is seen in patients with neurogenic communication disorders arising from stroke, traumatic brain injury, and degenerative neurological diseases. In perseveration, the patient appears to be stuck in a rigid mental set and cannot shift to an appropriate one. Kaplan, Gallagher, and Glosser (1998) consider perseveration an intrusive interference of previous responses and problematic for many aphasic patients.

Perseveration has been likened to a song that normal persons continue to process after the stimulus that prompted it has ceased. This occurrence in normal persons, however, is not as intense as what occurs in patients with neurogenic communication disorders and can be ceased relatively easily by distraction and shifts of attention.

Sandson and Albert (1984, p. 715) propose three types of perseveration: *stuck-in-set, recurrent,* and *continuous*:

> Stuck-in-set perseveration, the inappropriate maintenance of a current category or framework, involves an underlying process deficit in executive functioning and is related neuroanatomically to frontal lobe damage. Recurrent perseveration, the unintentional repetition of a previous response to a subsequent stimulus, involves an abnormal post-facilitation of memory traces and is related neuroanatomically to posterior left hemisphere damage. Continuous perseveration is the inappropriate prolongation or repetition of a behavior without interruption. It involves a deficit in motor output and is most common in patients with damage to the basal ganglia.

Perseveration behaviors typically occur in two modalities in patients with neurogenic communication disorders: verbal and graphic. An example of verbal perseveration is the patient repeating the same response to an initial question when others are asked (See Chapter 3). For example, in sentence completion therapy, the patient may respond to the request to complete the statement, "Red, white, and _____," with the correct verbal response: "Blue." The perseveration response occurs when the patient also responds with "Blue" to the following:

"Knife, fork, and _____," and "The United States of _____." According to Morganstein and Smith (2001, p. 388), perseveration can be highly problematic in therapy: "Typically, this tendency is discovered once treatment is underway and the clinician observes that the patient's responses, rather than demonstrating the advances in vocabulary retrieval and sentence use, contain recycled errors in word choice which are not evolving into something better." Graphic perseveration occurs when the patient's writing begins correctly, but then he or she repeats letters and often ends the writing attempt in a straight line.

Brain damage predisposes a person to perseveration by altering the brain's neurotransmitters, particularly the neuro-inhibitors. Psychologically, perseveration is a compulsive act and is perpetuated, at least in part, by the patient's obsessive need to maintain integrity of self. The verbal and graphic responses, incorrect though they may be, give the patient the appearance of normalcy. For the patient, an inappropriate response is better than no response; the patient does not want to feel or appear communicatively impotent. Perseveration can have significant negative effects on speech and language rehabilitation by reducing mental flexibility necessary for learning and adapting to the disability. It can also result in prolonged negative mental sets of anxiety, depression, hopelessness, and helplessness. Early initiation of treatment for patients with neurogenic communication disorders, especially for those with the tendency to perseverate, can counter habitual negative thoughts which may be developed by the patient without proper early intervention. By giving the patient abundant praise, support, and positive statements about his or her condition, the patient is likely to avoid contamination of negative thoughts due to perseveration.

The treatment of perseveration involves creating mental flexibility in the patient and can be incorporated into most speech and language therapies for neurogenic communication disorders. The objective is for the patient to develop a flexible mental set during the therapies and to improve his or her abilities to shift more rapidly and easily from one mental and behavior task to others. Instruction and encouragement are given to motivate the patient, and verbal rewards are provided, not simply for the correct responses, but for the patient's ability to shift from one mental set and behavior to another.

> Neuroscientists have not definitively linked perseveration to one particular damaged area of the brain.

Organic Depression-Anxiety Disorder

As discussed previously, patients with neurogenic communication disorders are predisposed to depression and anxiety. Upwards of 70% of persons with predominantly expressive nonfluent aphasia will experience depression-anxiety that is long lasting. Accurate incident and prevalence figures for depression and anxiety in patients with severe neurogenic communication disorders are unavailable due to the inability to get meaningful information about their mental and emotional states. This is particularly true for global aphasic patients.

The depression-anxiety disorder seen in many patients with neurogenic communication disorders can be reactive and a part of the grief response (See Chapter 10), primarily the result of a chemical imbalance caused by the brain injury, or a combination of both causal factors. Whereas reactive depression occurring in the grief response usually does not include significant anxiety, organic depression is often associated with "a feeling of impending doom." The angst felt by patients is a combination of despair and anxiety. Many patients become preoccupied and anxious with mental and body changes. Some patients may experience predominantly anxiety or depression in the organically-based depression-anxiety disorder and the predominance of one over the other may change over time. The anxiety component in depression-anxiety disorder may be based on the patient's concern about his or her depressive thoughts and unsuccessful attempts to avoid and escape them. In most patients, there is a loss of the *joie de vivre*, the carefree "joy of life" and pleasure in day-to-day living. With severe or chronic depression-anxiety, clinicians should be alert to indications of suicide and take immediate and appropriate prevention measures. The most important sign of suicide ideation is a report or indication from the patient, or his or her family, that suicide is being considered.

> Persons with anxiety disorders often have an underlying depression and anxiety is a frequent symptom of clinical depression.

When brain damage predisposes a patient to depression and anxiety, they primarily are a consequence of a neurochemical imbalance. In patients with neurogenic communication disorders, neurochemicals such as *serotonin* and *dopamine*, which are associated with "feelings of well-being," are out of balance for maintaining positive mood and emotion. Decreased serotonin, in particular, is linked to depression and anxiety disorders. However, there is always a psychological component to the etiology and persistence of depression-anxiety. The high incidence and prevalence of depression and anxiety in the expressive nonfluent aphasic person may be related to the frustrating nature of the communication disorder. Studies have shown a strong correlation and causal relationship between stress and depression-anxiety.

Counseling and antidepressant medication therapies are the two treatments for organic depression. Unfortunately, for many patients with neurogenic communication disorders, counseling, the "talking cure," is contraindicated. While counseling is important in a comprehensive treatment for anxiety-depression disorder in persons with normal communicative abilities, for many patients with neurogenic communication disorders, it is impractical because of the communication barrier. Patients with moderate to severe neurogenic communication disorders, especially those with aphasia, do not have the communication abilities to benefit from counseling. In addition, counseling with these patients may exacerbate their depression-anxiety because of the frustration they experience in being unable to communicate about the important issues brought up during the counseling sessions.

There are several antidepressant medications that effectively combat severe and prolonged anxiety-depression. Additionally, herbs and dietary supplements may also have a positive effect in improving general mood and in reducing mild-to-moderate depression and anxiety. While all drugs have side effects, most antidepressant medications are free from serious ones. Unfortunately, most antidepressants take several days and even weeks to begin to combat the depression-anxiety. In addition, physicians may try several different types and dosages of antidepressants medications before finding the optimal regimen. Of course, physicians rely on feedback from the patient about the ongoing effects of the medication and this feedback is not available from some patients with neurogenic communication disorders. In these circumstance, clinicians and family members can be valuable indirect sources of information about the patient's depression-anxiety and general mood. Especially with global aphasic patients, if there appears to be depression-anxiety, it is humane to recommend antidepressant medication therapy. Most antidepressant medications can be taken indefinitely with few if any side effects.

Anosognosia

Anosognosia is the denial of disease or disability in persons with brain injury. Denial is primarily a perceptual defense mechanism where the person blocks the reality of the situation from his or her conscious awareness. The denial may be complete with the patient refusing to perceive or accept the totality of the disease or disability. For example, a patient may not accept that a disordered limb is part of his or her body. Short-lived denial of hemiplegia occurs in more than half of patients with damage to the right hemisphere immediately after a stroke (Cutting, 1978). Carlat (1999) observes that extreme denial can be indications of psychotic thought processes. Benson and Ardila (1996) note that a patient with anosognosia may not see his or her disability in the proper perspective.

Some authorities limit the definition of anosognosia to "lack of awareness" of a disease or disability (Davis, 2007). However, active denial often co-occurs with lack of awareness especially in patients with visual neglect: "Denial of neglect and other deficits is characteristic of patients with neglect" (Myers, 2001). In addition, insufficient information about the nature and course of an illness or disability may simply cause lack of awareness. Therefore, in the discussion that follows, anosognosia will be broadly defined to be primarily denial of disease or disability.

Anosognosia may occur with all neurogenic communication disorders, but it plays an important role in fluent jargon aphasia associated with damage to the Wernicke's area and adjacent sites and tracts of the left temporal-parietal lobes. As reported in Chapter 3, Weinstein and Puig-Antich (1974) and Weinstein, Lyerly, Cole, and Ozer (1966) considered denial of disability as partially responsible for the persistent jargon in Wernicke's aphasia patients. In some, but not all fluent jargon aphasic patients, the meaningless speech is persistently produced when functional communication is obviously not taking place. A fluent jargon patient, for example, may utter a series of meaningless statements to a listener in an apparent attempt to obtain some good or service. There is clearly an attempt to express something important and meaningful. However, because the fluent jargon is incomprehensible to the listener, there is no consummation of the communicative act and consequently, no speaker satisfaction. However, because of anosognosia, many fluent jargon aphasic patients will continue to engage in the meaningless speech acts even though it is apparent that functional communication does not take place. Fluent jargon aphasic patients rarely pause for acknowledgment or engage in turn-taking in conversations (Owens, et al., 2000).

Many aphasic patients also act as if their jargon is perfectly normal and if the listener would only try harder to understand it, meaningful communication would take place. They are often irritated and angry with the listener's inability to understand their "perfectly normal" speech. A normal speaker would eventually see the futility of the fluent jargon for meaningful communication and stop speaking altogether despite the listener's inability to understand. The anger and irritation at the listener's inability to comprehend their fluent jargon is partially a result of the psychological defense mechanism of *projection*. Projection is attributing one's own intolerable wishes, thoughts, motivations, and feelings to another person.

The question may be asked, "Does fluent jargon have psychological meaning for the patient?" Of course, it is impossible accurately to generalize about the meaningless expressions produced by all aphasic patients. However, several possibilities exist for the psychological implications of jargon that go beyond denial and projection. First, fluent jargon may simply be a result of defective speech monitoring by the patient. Because of the receptive language disorder, the patient may be unable accurately to monitor his or her output. Consequently, the patient is unaware of the meaninglessness of the jargon and is essentially unaware that he or she is speaking abnormally. In effect, the patient perceives himself or herself as normal and others as abnormal. Second, psychologically, the jargon of the aphasic patient may be an attempt to maintain the integrity of self and the appearance of normal mental functions. By producing speech, albeit abnormal jargon, the patient maintains the illusion of normalcy and it is psychologically meaningful for his or her continuity of self. Third, the fluent jargon aphasic patient may be producing jargon because of damaged semantic processing, and the output is a reflection of his or her inner speech. The meaningless words and statements are meaningful to the patient and reflective of his or her cognitive processing. In this sense, it is a form of *idioglossia*, a private, distinctive language induced by brain damage.

> Prosopagnosia, sometimes called "face blindness," is a perceptual disorder where patients cannot recognize people by their faces. In one case, the patient could not recognize her children by their faces, but could identify them by their voices.

The treatment of anosognosia involves gradual and systematic confrontation of the disease or disability manifestations and symptom. This confrontation is done in a highly supportive and positive environment. If possible, the patient's family and friends should be present to offer support and encouragement. Never should the patient be brutally confronted with the reality of the disease or disability. Denial of disability serves as an important buffer to psychological pain, and less radical defenses should replace the patient's denial gradually and with support and encouragement. It should be remembered that although brain damage predisposes the patient to anosognosia, there is always a psychological consequence that goes beyond the neurological issues.

Homonymous Hemianopsia and Visual Neglect

Homonymous hemianopsia, a type of cortical or perceptual blindness, is the loss of vision in the same visual fields of both eyes. *Visual neglect*, which may occur with or without homonymous hemianopsia, involves the patient's inability and unwillingness to attend to one side of his or her body and environment. Patients with homonymous hemianopsia and visual neglect are sometimes said to have "lost of half their world."

When patients with neurogenic communication disorders have visual field disturbances, they typically have right homonymous hemianopsia with accompanying visual neglect of the right sides of their worlds. Severe visual field disturbance can affect reading, writing, and naming. Because of the patient's refusal or inability to cross midline during reading, he or she will only read the left side of a page with a consequent reduction in reading comprehension. When writing, the patient with right homonymous hemianopsia and visual neglect will not write beyond midline of a page. Similarly, when naming objects in the environment or in an array during testing, the patient will be compromised due to the visual field disturbances. In addition, some patients with homonymous hemianopsia and visual neglect will only consume food on one side of a plate, shave or apply makeup to one side of the face, and only attend to conversations occurring on one side of a room.

Homonymous hemianopsia and visual neglect are the result of central nervous system damage, often caused by stroke and traumatic brain injury, and both disorders also have a strong psychological component. Psychologically, a partial explanation for the patient neglecting one side of the visual word is that unwanted physical changes have occurred on the affected side of his or her body. The hemiplegia threatens the patient's integrity of self and sense of wholeness. The visual neglect is partially a consequence of the coping style and psychological defense of *avoidance*. By avoiding the negatively affected side of his or her world, the patient is partially and temporarily protected from anxiety and negative emotions.

The treatment for homonymous hemianopsia involves gradual and systematic exercises designed to confront the affected side and cross midline. These therapies can occur during reading, writing, objecting naming exercises, and during conversations held in the patient's room. If the patient also has *dysphagia*, a swallowing disorder, crossing midline during eating can also be a goal of therapy. Attempts by the patient to confront the negativity associated with the disordered side of his or her world should be encouraged in an accepting environment, and each attempt to cross midline immediately praised and rewarded.

> According to Culbertson (2009), in the case of hemianopsia, if opposite halves of the visual field are involved for each eye, the hemianopsia is *heteronymous.*

Euphoria

Euphoria, an elevated mood and heightened sense of well-being, occurs in normal persons but also from anoxia. According to Craig and Cummings (1995), euphoria can be a chronic condition in fluent jargon aphasic patients. In normal persons, euphoric episodes result from intensely exciting and pleasurable experiences, such as those involving love, sex, and religious experiences. It is interesting to note that in certain religious ceremonies where participants report euphoria, they often talk in "tongues," which has many similarities to aphasic jargon.

Denial may also result in euphoria. Denial, a radical perceptual defense discussed in Chapter 9, blocks the reality of the situation from the patient's consciousness leaving him or her with only positive thoughts and emotions. Ritchie (1961, pp. 35-36) observed: "I heeded only the most obvious optimistic things that were said to me and for the rest I did not hear them or came to the conclusion that they were wrong. If I had allowed myself to be given a glimpse of the truth, I believe I would have gone out of my mind."

Should euphoria in the patient with neurogenic communication disorders be considered a negative rehabilitative and prognostic factor and treated as a maladjustment to the disability? There are two issues regarding chronic euphoria in individuals with neurogenic communication disorders. First, the patient with euphoria has little anxiety about his or her disability and often seems unconcerned and even content with the predicament. Because the euphoric patient is unrealistic about his or her communication disorder, it can be considered a psychological maladjustment. The patient with persistent euphoria does not appreciate the reality of his or her situation. Although it appears that the euphoric patient has accepted his or her predicament, he or she is experiencing inappropriate and maladaptive emotions about it. Dissatisfaction with the status quo are primary motivators for patients to improve in rehabilitation, and euphoric patients lack this necessary ingredient to improve.

> In flight training, pilots are taught that euphoria, an elevated mood and heightened sense of well-being, are an indication of oxygen deprivation at high altitudes.

The second issue about euphoria in the patient with neurogenic communication disorders involves the fact that there are few if any realistic treatments. It would seem inhumane to attempt to reduce or eliminate a patient's elevated mood and heightened sense of well-being. While the overriding goal may be to increase the patient's motivation and willingness to participate in rehabilitation, attempting to reduce or eliminate the patient's euphoria is not a realistic therapeutic objective. However, gradual confrontation of the patient to his or her disabilities and predicament in a supportive and positive environment may cause him or her to see the need to participate in rehabilitation.

Maladaptive Behavior

Although all patients with neurogenic communication disorders may exhibit behavioral problems, Wernicke aphasia and traumatic brain injured patients often have significant behavioral issues affecting rehabilitation. Benson and Ardila (1996, p. 141) report that behavioral problems in Wernicke aphasia patients are often dramatic: "Wernicke aphasia patients often misinterpret their own problems and suspect that family members, friends, doctors, nursing staff, and others are the real cause of their comprehension difficulty. They accuse others of not listening carefully or of speaking in a code; this can lead to a suspicious, paranoid attitude producing an agitated, even dangerous behavior." As discussed in Chapter 7, the behavioral problems in individuals with traumatic brain injuries can be divided into hyperfunctional and hypofunctional disorders.

Hyperfunctional disorders include hypersexuality, aggressiveness, mood swings, impulsiveness, increased socialness, euphoria, increased attentiveness, and restlessness. Patients with hyperfunctional disorders appear unable to refrain and restrain excessive behaviors. Hypofunctional disorders include hyposexuality, apathy, reduced spontaneity, decreased socialness, depression, decreased attentiveness, and psychomotor retardation. Patients with hypofunctional behavioral disturbances seem to lack energy and have lost the will to engage in day-to-day activities. While all of the above behavioral disorders may occur in people without brain injury, neurological insult can predispose patients with neurogenic communication disorder to them.

Ylvisaker, Szekeres, and Feeney (2001) note that behavioral and psychosocial difficulties may be a result of the traumatic brain injury, but they are often complicated by preinjury challenges and post injury adjustment problems. "Our work with several hundred adolescents and young adults with chronic school and work problems and general community reintegration difficulty suggests that behavioral and psychosocial themes are often at the core of these problems, although in most cases complex patterns of interaction exist between cognition and behavioral consequences of the injury" (Ylvisaker, Szekeres, and Feeney, 2001, p. 777).

> Patients who make frequent commanding, ordering, and demanding statements may be feeling confused and disoriented, and their behaviors are attempts to take control of their lives.

As discussed in Chapter 7, improvement of the patient's mental executive functioning (metacognition) is a primary long-term rehabilitation goal in persons with traumatic brain injury. The rehabilitation team works cooperatively to manage the adjustment problems of the patient with particular emphasis on the risk factors associated with the patient's discharge to home. The same primary long-term rehabilitation goal is applied to Wernicke aphasia patients predisposed to paranoid ideation or dangerous behaviors. Table 8.2 lists, describes, and provides the psycho-organic maladaptive reactions in neurogenic communication disorders.

Table 8.2: Psycho-Organic Maladaptive Reactions in Neurogenic Communication Disorders

Psychological Reaction	Description	Rehabilitation Objectives
Emotional Lability	Involuntary, exaggerated emotionality	Reduce or eliminate the predisposing, precipitating, and perpetuating factors
Catastrophic Reaction	Psychobiological breakdown; panic attack	Prevention and minimization
Perseveration	Inappropriate continuation of an act and mental set	Mental flexibility
Organic Depression-Anxiety Disorder	Organically-based depression and anxiety	Environmental manipulation, counseling, antidepressant medication
Anosognosia	Denial of disease or disability	Gradual and systematic confrontation of the disease or disability manifestations and symptom
Homonymous Hemianopsia and Visual Neglect	Cortical or perceptual blindness	Gradual and systematic exercises to confront the affected side and cross midline
Euphoria	Elevated mood and heightened sense of well-being	Gradual confrontation of the patient to his or her disabilities and predicament
Maladaptive Behavior	Hyperfunctional and hypofunctional behavior disorders; paranoia	Improvement of mental executive functioning (metacognition)

Chapter Summary

Some patients with neurogenic communication disorders are predisposed to psychological dysfunction and maladaptive behavior because of the nature, type, and location of the brain injury. Exaggerated emotionality, catastrophic reactions, and perseveration occur in some patients resulting in excessive crying, panic attacks, and the impaired ability to shift mentally. A large percentage of patients with neurogenic communication disorders also suffer depression and anxiety that are long lasting. Brain damage can also predispose a patient to denial of disability and visual neglect. Wernicke aphasia and traumatic brain injured patients may also have psycho-organically based maladaptive behaviors.

Study and Discussion Questions

1. What are the multiple determinants of the psychology of neurogenic communication disorders?

2. What are the "medical" and "social" models regarding the psychology of neurogenic communication disorders?

3. Draw a human brain and identify the likely sites of damage and their corresponding psychological reactions.

4. Is emotional lability an exaggerated or inappropriate emotional response? Explain the difference.

5. Why are catastrophic reactions considered "psychobiological breakdowns?"

6. Discuss how echolalia and perseveration are related.

7. Why are depression and anxiety co-occurring states in many patients with predominantly expressive nonfluent aphasia?

8. Describe anosognosia.

9. Compare and contrast homonymous hemianopsia and visual neglect.

10. What are your thoughts about euphoria that occurs in some patients with neurogenic communication disorders?

Is euphoria a positive or negative prognostic indicator?
Explain your answer.

11. Compare and contrast hyperfunctional and hypofunctional
behavioral disorders seen in some patients with neurogenic
communication disorders.

References

Benson, F. D. and Ardila, A. (1996). *Aphasia: A clinical perspective.*
New York: Oxford University Press.

Black, F. (1975). Unilateral brain lesions and MMPI performance: A
preliminary study. *Perceptual and Motor Skills*, 40: 87-93.

Carlat, D. (1999). *The psychiatric interview.* Philadelphia: Lippincott,
Williams & Wilkins.

Carota, A., Rossetti, A, Karapanayiotides, T, and Bogousslavsky, J.
(2001). Catastrophic reaction in acute stroke: A reflex behavior in
aphasic patients. *Neurology*, 57:1902-1905.

Craig, A. and Cummings, J. (1995). Neuropsychiatric aspects of
aphasia. In *Handbook of neurological speech and language disorders,*
H. Kirshner (Ed.). New York: Marcel Dekker, Inc.

Culbertson, W.R. (2009). *Speech and hearing anatomy and physiology*
(in press). San Diego: Plural Publishing.

Cummings, J.L., Arciniegas, D.B., Brooks, B.R., Herndon, R.M.,
Lauterbach, E.C., Pioro, E.P., Robinson, R.G., Scharre, D.W., Schiffer,
R.B., Weintraub, D. (2006). Defining and diagnosing involuntary
emotional expression disorder. *CNS Spectrums.* 2006 Jun;11(6):1-7.

Cutting, J. (1978). Study of anosognosia. *Journal of Neurology,
Neurosurgery and Psychiatry*, 41, 548-555.

Davis, G.A. (2007). *Aphasiology: Disorders and clinical practice* (2nd ed.) Boston: Pearson, Allyn and Bacon.

Duffy, J.R. (2005). *Motor speech disorders: Substrates, differential diagnosis, and management* (2nd ed.). St. Louis: Mosby.

Eisenson, J. (1984). *Adult aphasia*, (2nd ed.). Englewood Cliffs, NJ: Prentice-Hall.

Frank, C. (1998). Overview of psychiatric disease for the speech-language practitioner. In *Medical speech-language pathology: A practitioner's guide.* A. Johnson and B. Jacobson (Eds). New York: Thieme.

Gainotti, G. (1972). Emotional behavior and hemisphere side of the lesion. *Cortex*, 8: 41-55.

Gainotti, G. (1989). The meaning of emotional disturbances resulting from unilateral brain injury. In *Emotions and the dual brain,* G. Gainotti, and C. Caltagirone (Eds). New York: Springer-Verlag.

Gasparini, W., Satz, P., Heilman, K., and Coolidge, F. (1978). Hemispheric asymmetries of affective processing as determined by the Minnesota Multiphasic Personality Inventory. *Journal of Neurology, Neurosurgery and Psychiatry*, 41: 470-473.

Gordon, W., Hibbard, M., Egelko, S., and Diller, L. (1985). The multifaceted nature of the cognitive deficits following stroke: Unexpected findings. *Archives of Physical Medicine and Rehabilitation*, 66: 338.

Gordon, W., Hibbard, M., and Morganstein, S. (1996). Response to Tanner and Gerstenberger. In *Forums in Clinical Aphasiology*, C. Code (Ed). London, UK: Whurr Publishers.

Kaplan, E., Gallagher, R.E., and Glosser, G. (1998). Aphasia-related disorders. In *Acquired aphasia* (3rd ed.). M. Sarno (Ed). San Diego: Academic Press.

Katz, I.R. (2000). Agitation, aggressive behavior, and catastrophic reaction. *International Psychogeriatrics*, 12: 119-123 Cambridge University Press.

Laraia, M. (1998). Biological context of psychiatric nursing care. In *principles and practice of psychiatric nursing (*6th Ed.). G. Stuart and M. Laraia (Eds), St. Louis: Mosby.

Lipsey, J., Spencer, W., Rabins, P., and Robinson, R. (1986). Phenomenological comparison of poststroke depression and functional depression. *American Journal of Psychiatry*, 143:4.

Meyers, P.S. (2001). Communication disorders associated with right hemisphere damage. In *Language intervention strategies in aphasia and related neurogenic communication disorders* (4th ed.), R. Chapey, (Ed). Philadelphia: Lippincott Williams & Wilkins.

Morganstein, S. and Smith, M. (2001). Thematic language stimulation therapy. In *Language intervention strategies in aphasia and related neurogenic communication disorders* (4th ed.), R. Chapey, (Ed). Philadelphia: Lippincott Williams & Wilkins.

Owens, R., Metz, D., and Haas, A. (2000). *Introduction to Communication Disorders.* Boston: Allyn & Bacon.

Robinson, R., and Benson, D. (1981). Depression in aphasic patients: Frequency, severity, and clinical-pathological correlations. *Brain and Language*, 14: 282-291.

Robinson, R., Lipsey, J., Bolla-Wilson, K, Bolduc, P., Pearlson, G, Rao, K., and Price, T. (1985). Mood disorders in left-handed stroke patients. *American Journal of Psychiatry*, 142:12.

Robinson, R., Boston, J., Starkstein, S. and Price, T. (1988). Comparison of mania and depression after brain injury: Causal factors. *American Journal of Psychiatry*, 145:2.

Robinson, R. (1986). *Depression and stroke*. Psychiatric Annals, 17(11): 731-740.

Sackeim, H., Greenberg, M., Weiman, A., Gur, R., Hungerbahler, J., and Geschwin, N. (1982). Hemispheric asymmetry in the expression of positive and negative emotions: Neurological evidence. *Archives of Neurology*, 39: 210-218.

Sackeim, H. and Weber, S. (1982). Functional brain asymmetry in the regulation of emotion: Implications for bodily manifestations of stress. In *Handbook of stress*, L. Goldberger and S. Breznitz (Eds). New York: Macmillan.

Sandson J. and Albert, M. (1984). Varieties of perseveration. *Neuropsychologia*, 22(6):715-32.

Scoppetta, M., Di Gennaro, G., and Scoppetta C. (2005). Selective serotonin reuptake inhibitors prevent emotional lability in healthy subjects. *Eur Rev Med Pharmacol Science*, (6):343-8.

Smeltzer, D., Nasrallah, H., and Miller, S. (1994). Psychotic disorders. In J. Silver, S. Yudofsky, and R. Hales (Eds.) *Neuropsychiatry of traumatic brain injury*. Washington, DC: American Psychiatric Press.

Tanner, D. and Gerstenberger, D. (1996). Clinical forum 9: The grief model in aphasia. In *Forums in Clinical Aphasiology*, C. Code (Ed). London: Whurr Publishers

Tanner, D. (2003, Winter). Eclectic perspectives on the psychology of aphasia. *J. Allied Health: 32:256-260.*

Tanner, D. (2007). *The medical-legal and forensic aspects of communication disorders, voice prints, and speaker profiling.* Tucson: Lawyers and Judges Publishing Company.

Tanner, D. (2009). *The psychology of neurogenic communication disorders: A primer for health care professionals.* New York: iUniverse.

Tardiff, K. (1997). Evaluation and treatment of violent patients. In D. Stoff, J. Breiling, and J.D. Maser (Eds). *Handbook of antisocial behavior* (pp. 445-453). New York: John Wiley & Sons.

Tetnowski, J. A. (2003). Foreword. In D. Tanner, *The psychology of neurogenic communication disorders: A primer for health care professionals.* Boston: Allyn and Bacon.

Weinstein, E., Lyerly, O., Cole, M., and Ozer, M. (1966). Meaning in jargon aphasia. *Cortex*, 2: 165-187.

Weinstein, E. and Puig-Antich, J. (1974). Jargon and its analogues. *Cortex*, 10:75-83.

Williams, W. Evans, J., Fleminger, S. (2003). Neurorehabilitation and cognitive-behaviour therapy of anxiety disorders after brain injury: An overview and a case illustration of obsessive-compulsive disorder. *Neuropsychological Rehabilitation*, Volume 13, Issues 1 & 2:133 -148.

Ylvisaker, M., Szekeres, S.F., and Feeney, T. (2001). Communication disorders associated with traumatic brain injury. In *Language intervention strategies in aphasia and related neurogenic communication disorders* (4th ed.), R. Chapey, (Ed). Philadelphia: Lippincott Williams & Wilkins.

Chapter Nine: Defense Mechanisms and Coping Styles

"Sometimes a cigar is just a cigar."

Sigmund Freud

Chapter Preview: This chapter examines the role defense mechanisms and coping styles play in the psychological adjustment to neurogenic communication disorders. Avoidance, ego restriction, physical escape, and autistic fantasy are discussed as ways patients may cope with threats of a predominantly external nature. Psychological defense mechanisms and coping styles available to language-deprived patients for threats of a predominantly internal nature are discussed including denial, repression, psychological regression, passive-aggression, reaction formation, altruism, sublimation, substitution, displacement and projection, and dissociation. Psychological defense mechanisms and coping styles compromised by the loss of language are reviewed including rationalization and intellectualization, suppression, undoing, and humor.

Defense Mechanisms and Coping Styles

Defense mechanisms are ways humans protect themselves from full awareness of distressing feelings, thoughts, and desires. Porcerelli, Thomas, Hibbard, and Cogan (1998) note that the concept of ego defense mechanisms has stood the test of time and provides important information about normal development, psychopathology, and adaptation. All people use defense mechanisms to cope with reality, protect themselves from anxiety, and to exclude disturbing thoughts from consciousness. Defense mechanisms are important for individuals to maintain *self-esteem*. Self-esteem is a personal judgment of worth based on a self-ideal (Stuart, 2001a).

According to Porcerelli and Hibbard (2004, p. 466), Sigmund Freud introduced the concept of defense mechanisms in 1894: "He conceptualized defenses as mental forces that opposed unacceptable ideas or feelings that, if acknowledged, would cause significant distress." Anna Freud, in *The Ego and the Mechanisms of Defense*, expanded the concept of defense mechanisms and suggested classification systems (A. Freud, 1936). Wallerstein (1999) notes that defense mechanisms are hypothetical constructs denoting the way the mind functions. Carlat (1999) considers coping styles and defense mechanisms similar concepts. While defense mechanisms and coping styles play an important explanatory role in contemporary mental health (Boyd, 1998), there is little agreement about them and much overlap (Stuart and Laraia, 1998).

Generally, psychological defense mechanisms and coping styles can be placed on a continuum of adaptability ranging from mature and adaptive to those that are immature, maladaptive, neurotic, and radical attempts to cope with stressors. Immature, maladaptive, neurotic, and radical psychological defense mechanisms and coping styles are used when stressors, and the individual's ability to cope with them, become overwhelming. Wallerstein (1999, p. 59) observes: "Defenses or defensive behaviors can be viewed as complexly *layered* and, depending on whether the perspective is 'upward' syntonic and conscious or 'downward' toward the more archaic (infantile) and unconscious, can be seen to serve impulsive discharge pressures in relation to the higher psychic layerings or defensive avoidant needs in relation to the lower psychic layerings."

Anna Freud (1895-1982), Sigmund Freud's daughter continued his work regarding psychoanalysis. She discovered several defense mechanisms and coping styles.

Unfortunately, in the psychology and psychiatric literature on psychological defense mechanisms and coping styles, there is no consensus on the nature and adjustment value of each psychological defense mechanism and coping style. In addition, the use of a particular psychological defense mechanism and coping style, and its productive contribution to mental health, is also dependent on the nature of the stressor and how extensively and appropriately it is used. Even a mature defense mechanism and coping style can be maladaptive when used inappropriately. However, it is generally accepted that the mechanisms of psychological defenses are subconscious, their behaviors are conscious and observable. Wallerstein (1999) notes that because defense mechanisms are theoretical abstractions, it is irrelevant whether they are conscious or subconscious. (In this text, "unconscious" refers to loss of consciousness because of brain damage and "subconscious" refers to thought processes, drives, and emotions below the person's conscious awareness).

Defense mechanisms and coping styles are important to understanding neurogenic communication disorders for two reasons. First, defense mechanisms and coping styles play an important role in the psychological adaptation to disabilities. They affect the symptoms of neurogenic communication disorders and treatment efficacy. Second, in language-deprived aphasic patients, only nonverbal defense mechanisms may be available for coping and adjustment to the disability (Tanner, 2009). Patients without language, global aphasics, have special adjustment issues not experienced by persons with normal language functions. Even in aphasic patients with partial language, the utilization of verbal defense mechanisms and coping styles may be impaired or less accessible.

In the discussion that follows, several psychological defenses and coping styles will be reviewed relative their application to patients with neurogenic communication disorders and the likelihood of being utilized by language-deprived persons. It is acknowledged that some of the psychological defenses and coping styles discussed below are controversial concerning their definitions and adaptation value. However, it is necessary to review possible ways patients with neurogenic communication disorders may attempt to adjust to their disabilities and cope with the limitations caused by them.

Avoidance and Escape from Predominantly External Threats

Defense mechanisms and coping styles are patterned thoughts, feelings, reactions, and behaviors that arise in response to perceived or real internal or external threats. Usually, they are subconscious and occur as an involuntary response. When the perceived threats and dangers are primarily prompted by an internal thought or memory, the defense mechanism and coping style depend on avoidance of this thought or memory (Chisholm, 1993). Perceived threats and dangers that are primarily internal in nature, and the defense mechanisms and coping styles used to deal with them, are difficult to discover and understand in many patients with neurogenic communication disorders because of the communication barriers. When the perceived threats and dangers are primarily prompted by external threats and dangers, the defense mechanisms and coping styles involve avoidance and physical escape from specific situations and environments. The primary defense mechanisms and coping styles relevant to patients with neurogenic communication disorders used to deal with threats of an external nature are avoidance, ego restriction, physical escape, and autistic fantasy.

Avoidance

Avoidance is a basic and innate defense mechanism and coping style. When a person is confronted with unpleasantness, he or she can simply try to avoid it. It is often used when a person is confronted with an external threat although avoidance of disturbing thoughts lies at the core of many defense mechanisms and coping styles. The avoiding person may be preoccupied with thoughts of rejection (Carlat, 1999).

There are two aspects to avoidance: *postponement* and *refusal*. In postponement, the avoiding person delays confronting the anxiety provoking situation or thought which provides temporary relief. The refusing person declines confronting the distressing and anxiety provoking stimulus often after repeated postponements. The extreme use of avoidance creates the *avoidant personality disorder*: "These patients experience few positive reinforcers from self or others, are relentlessly vigilant and on guard, and are quick to distance themselves from anxious anticipation of life's painful and negatively reinforcing experiences" (Millon and Meagher, 2004, p. 109). In patients with neurogenic communication disorders, avoidance as a defense mechanism and coping style may be misunderstood and inappropriately addressed during evaluation and treatment.

In persons with neurogenic communication disorders, there is much to avoid. Many patients must undergo painful therapies and invasive diagnostic procedures. The very nature of many therapies require the patient to confront his or her disabilities, often with little time to prepare psychologically. This is particularly true concerning speech and language therapies because awareness of errors and monitoring of them are essential treatment objectives. Another major negative consequence of neurogenic communication disorders prompting the avoidance defense mechanism and coping style is confinement to a medical facility with new demands, routines, and often a total lack of privacy. There are also the costs of the medical care and the neurogenic communication disorder's implications on the patient's future employment and quality of life.

The use of avoidance as a defense mechanism and coping style should be understood, permitted, and in some cases encouraged. When used appropriately and sparingly, this defense mechanism and coping style can provide necessary relief from the negativity and stress associated with the neurogenic communication disorder. For many patients, attempts to postpone or refuse diagnostic procedures and treatments are necessary and adaptive ways of coping with the neurogenic communication disorder.

Efforts should be taken to encourage the avoiding patient to participate fully in the rehabilitation program by providing support, counseling, and gradual confrontation with stressful and negative aspects of the neurogenic communication disorder. However, ultimately it is the patient's prerogative to decide whether he or she participates in rehabilitation, when, and to what extent. While many patients with neurogenic communication disorders cannot express their rationale for using avoidance, this defense mechanism and coping style should be understood, tolerated, and respected. By doing so, health care professionals, family, and friends of the patient ultimately increase the likelihood that the patient with a neurogenic communication disorders will eventually be optimally motivated to participate in rehabilitation.

> Avoidance is the simplest know defense mechanism and coping style.

The avoidance defense mechanism and coping style does not require language to be effectively used. Consequently, language-deprived patients can avoid threatening and unpleasant situations and related thoughts by engaging in avoidance. When used sparingly, postponement and refusal can be adaptive ways of coping with the stressors associated with neurogenic communication disorders which deprive the patient of language. For global aphasic patients, the avoidance defense mechanism and coping style may be one of few ways of finding relief from the negativity and unpleasantness associated with communication disorders.

Ego Restriction

Anna Freud first identified the defense mechanism and coping style of *ego restriction* (Mahl, 1971). In ego restriction, a type of avoidance, a person abandons an activity in response to anxiety. In the extreme, the individual voluntarily gives up an entire area of ego involvement rather than to risk the possibility of not succeeding at it. The anxiety is based on threats to self-esteem.

Patients with neurogenic communication disorders, like many persons with brain damage, are subject to reductions in self-esteem (Wepman, 1962). The knowledge that they have suffered brain damage threatens their self-concept and can reduce their self-esteem. Patients with neurogenic communication disorders face the reality that they cannot perform many day-to-day activities as well as they did previously. Additionally, many patients are aware that others, including health care professionals, are analyzing and judging their behaviors and actions. Neurogenic communication disorders are fertile grounds for questions regarding mental and physical competence and consequent reductions in self-esteem.

Patient with neurogenic communication disorders, including global aphasics, may display ego restriction in employment, family roles, social activities, and concerning rehabilitation. In employment, a patient may abandon an aspect of an occupation or even an entire vocation because of ego restriction. The patient's abandonment of an employment activity is not due to realistic inabilities to perform them due to the neurogenic communication disorder, it is a result of anxiety associated with the threat to self-esteem should he or she fail. He or she may also similarly abandon an important family function, such as taking a leadership role in purchasing issues. Ego restriction may be seen in social activities, especially those requiring extensive communication. In rehabilitation, a patient may abandon the role of a willing and motivated patient, not because he or she has a poor prognosis, but because the potential of failure provokes unacceptable levels of anxiety.

Physical Escape

Carson, et al. (1988) observe that when avoidance is impractical or impossible, it may be necessary for a person to physically *escape* a negative and threatening situation thereby providing psychological relief. Like avoidance, escape is an innate and basic defense mechanism and coping style providing immediate relief from anxiety. In patients with neurogenic communication disorders, the psychological need to physically escape from negative and threatening thoughts and situations may occur during evaluations and therapies. Patients with functional speech and language can report their need to escape a particular negative and threatening situation. They may say, "This is a stressful therapy, can we take a break?" and "Let's take a breather from this therapy and do something else now." Patients without functional speech and language may show their need to physical escape through fidgeting, agitation, and distraction.

Physical escape is observed in patients with neurogenic communication disorders confronted with external threats, but like avoidance, the need to escape from disturbing thoughts lies at the core of many defense mechanisms and coping styles. Eisenson (1984) notes that a catastrophic reaction (See Chapter 8) is a psychobiological breakdown, which in the extreme, may result in the patient losing consciousness. Because the catastrophic reaction is based on the need to fight or flee from a perceived threat, a patient's loss of consciousness can be considered, at least psychologically, the ultimate escape. By losing consciousness, the patient escapes from the external threat of the situation and the accompanying threatening thoughts.

Patients with neurogenic communication disorders may disguise their reasons to escape from threatening therapeutic situations by feigning the need to go to the bathroom, wanting to return to their room for clothing or objects, illness, and so forth. Especially in patients with nonfunctional speech and language abilities, these disguised reasons for escaping from threatening therapeutic situations may only involve nonverbal indications of distress by the patient. Of course, this is not to say that all nonverbal requests by patients with nonfunctional speech and language abilities to stop a therapy and do something else are based on the escape psychological defense mechanism and coping style. However, escape from threatening a therapeutic situation should be considered especially in patients with adjustment challenges. Like avoidance, escape should be understood, permitted, and sometimes encouraged. This defense mechanism and coping style can provide necessary relief from the negativity and stress associated with the neurogenic communication disorder.

> Freud believed that humans have only two
> drives: sex and aggression.

Global aphasic patients, those individuals with neurogenic communication disorders who are deprived of language, can use escape as an adaptive defense mechanism and coping style. Under most circumstances, language is not necessary to escape from unpleasantness. The patient may show nonverbal indications for the need to escape including fidgeting, distraction, and physical attempts to leave a particular stressful situation. When used sparingly, global aphasic patients can find relief from negativity and unpleasantness associated with their communication disorders by engaging in the psychological defense and coping style of escape.

Autistic Fantasy

Autistic fantasy is a form of escape through daydreaming and a symbolic way of meeting psychological needs. It is excessive daydreaming as a substitute for more appropriate action to deal with emotional conflicts (Burgess and Clements, 1998). During fantasy escape, the individual protects and supports the ego and symbolically deals with emotional conflicts (Carson, et al., 1988). Typical fantasy escapes include daydreaming about occupational, athletic, sexual, financial, and social activities. (This discussion does not address subconscious fantasies). The retreat into a fantasy world is considered an immature defense mechanism and coping style, but for patients with neurogenic communication disorders, it can be desirable, mature, and adaptive given the extreme circumstances. For normal persons, the fantasy defense mechanism and coping style, when used in excess, can be socially undesirable, but it can bridge the gap between desire and reality for patients with neurogenic communication disorders. It can help them obtain needed relief from social and communicative frustrations in their retreat into imaginary worlds.

Patients engaging in autistic fantasy escape may be misdiagnosed as distracted, "blanking out," unresponsive, and unmotivated in rehabilitation. While it is true that some patients with neurogenic communication disorders may be unmotivated and have attention disorders, especially those with traumatic brain injury, others may be escaping reality as an attempt to cope with psychological distress. Rather than being disengaged from a particular therapy because of neurological deficits, the patient may be withdrawing and daydreaming as a symbolic way of meeting his or her psychological needs. The patient may be dealing with emotional conflicts and experiencing a brief respite from the ego threats associated with confronting the disability in therapy. Of course, the use of fantasy escape by persons with neurogenic communication disorders can also be maladaptive, socially undesirable, and interfere with optimal speech and language rehabilitation. If the patient frequently avoids therapies and social interaction by engaging in fantasy escape, he or she will not benefit optimally from rehabilitation.

Normal persons engage in autistic fantasy escapes use visual imagery facilitated by internal monologues. Global aphasia patients, because of the language deprivation, are limited to visual imagery during fantasy escapes. However, the psychological defense mechanism and coping style of autistic fantasy can be successfully employed by language-deprived patients to satisfy their psychological needs. Table 9.1 shows avoidance and escape defense mechanisms and coping styles from predominantly external threats and stressors.

Table 9.1: Avoidance and Escape Defense Mechanisms and Coping Styles from Predominantly External Threats and Stressors.

Psychological Defense and Coping Style	Description	Use by Language-Deprived Patient
Avoidance	Simple avoidance of perceived external threat	Yes
Ego Restriction	Abandonment of an activity in response to anxiety and threats to self-esteem	Yes
Physical Escape	Physical escape from a negative and threatening situation	Yes
Autistic Fantasy	Escape through daydreaming as a symbolic way of meeting psychological needs	Yes

Psychological Defense Mechanisms and Coping Styles for Predominantly Internal Threats and Stressors

It is acknowledged that there is no clear distinction between threats of an external and internal nature because perceived external dangers are also accompanied by the thoughts related to them. However, this distinction is appropriate when discussing patients with neurogenic communication disorders because discovery and analysis of perceived threats and dangers are hindered because of the communication barriers. As noted above, when the perceived threats and dangers are primarily prompted by internal thoughts or memories, the defense mechanism and coping style involve denial, avoidance, or some other way of blocking, suppressing, or repressing them. The following defense mechanisms and coping styles are relevant to patients with neurogenic communication disorders, and most are at least partially available to language-deprived, global aphasic persons.

Denial

In Chapter 8, anosognosia was defined as the denial of disease or disability as a consequence of brain injury. However, denial is integral to many defense mechanisms and coping styles that do not result from brain damage. Denial can be organically based, as discussed in the previous chapter, but also occur as the initial stage in the grief response (See Chapter 10). Denial as a defense mechanism and coping style protects the ego, reduces anxiety, and keeps unacceptable thoughts and feelings from conscious awareness.

> People with substance abuse problems often deny the problems.

Authorities on denial as a defense mechanism and coping style sometimes make a distinction between complete and partial denial. In partial denial, the person may acknowledge some aspects of reality while minimizing them. However, partial denial is more likely the activation, at least partially, of rationalization, intellectualization, or other defense mechanisms and coping styles to deal with psychological threats. Denial protects the ego by blocking from conscious awareness threatening and unpleasant events and situations. It is considered a perceptual defense mechanism and coping style not requiring language. As such, it is a natural and likely defense utilized by language-deprived individuals

Denial can be an effective tool to delay confrontation with psychological threats for patients without language. However, persistent use of denial is a negative prognostic factor for optimal speech and language rehabilitation. Patients persistently engaged in denial are unrealistic and may never fully confront their disabilities. This negates many of the benefits of therapy and other treatments. Denial is a radical defense requiring substantial energy by the denying person to maintain it. It takes extensive psychological energy to deny some aspect of reality in the presence of clear evidence of its existence.

Denying patients also may negatively affect the rehabilitation team. Because the patient does not believe he or she has a communication disorder, or other disability related to the neurological event, some rehabilitation team members may feel useless to perform their duties. Their professional roles are threatened when a patient clearly in need of rehabilitation denies his or her disability and refuses treatment. Unfortunately, some rehabilitation professionals brutally confront the denying patient with the reality of his or her situation. In most cases, this is counterproductive often causing the patient to be more fixed and rigid in his or her denial.

Repression

Repression differs from suppression in that the former is done automatically and involuntarily. Many defense mechanisms and coping styles are manifestations of repression. In repression, negative thoughts, feelings, drives, memories, and ideas are excluded from consciousness by inhibiting them before or after they reach a conscious level. In repression, they are detected and stored, but recall is inhibited (See Chapter 7). Thus, negative thoughts, feelings, drives, memories, and ideas are inaccessible preventing unbearable anxiety.

Repression may be one factor in the amnesia surrounding the cerebral insult experienced by many patients with neurogenic communication disorders. Many patients cannot remember the events immediately co-occurring with the stroke or traumatic brain injury. For example, they do not remember the car accident or collapsing to the floor with a stroke. While brain damage, particularly to the hippocampus, may be the physical basis for the post-traumatic or post stroke selective amnesia, repression of the events surrounding the catastrophe can also contribute or account for the memory loss. Carlat (1999) considers repression a way of forcing the emotion out of conscious awareness.

Brain damage may also undo repression and cause the patient to experience anxiety because previously repressed memories surface. For example, a traumatic brain injured patient may experience anxiety because he or she is unable to keep repressed painful thoughts about childhood from conscious awareness. This *return of the repressed* can account from some anxious behaviors seen in patients with severe traumatic brain injuries and strokes.

Psychotherapy, the "talking cure," addresses the failure of repression to prevent conscious awareness of negative thoughts, feelings, drives, memories, and ideas. Using the person's intact reasoning abilities and unimpaired memory, psychotherapists help critically to analyze the repressed. The goal is to have the conscious ego examine the repressed information logically and maturely. Unfortunately, most patients with aphasia cannot benefit from psychotherapy due to the communication disorder and because aphasia causes a loss of abstract attitude (See Chapter 2). An abstract attitude is necessary to reason and critically analyze issues related to repression. Traumatic brain injured patients may also lack the mental executive functioning necessary to benefit from psychotherapy. Repression is well within the range of aphasic and traumatic brain injured patients, but psychotherapy to treat repressional dysfunctions is contraindicated for many patients with neurogenic communication disorders.

> Some authorities believe "slips of the tongue" are the surfacing of subconscious repressed memories.

Psychological Regression

Stuart (2001b) describes *psychological regression* as a retreat to a more secure and comfortable level of adjustment. The patient engaged in regression as a defense mechanism and coping style returns to a level of reaction to life's stressors that he or she has outgrown. It is usually a subconscious return to an immature stage of psychological adjustment to avoid anxiety and involves thoughts, behaviors, and emotions. Chapman (1976, p. 63) provides an example of total regression occurring in a woman who finds problems of marriage and child rearing overwhelmingly stressful: "She may flee into psychogenic physical symptoms that allow her to become a dependent, childlike invalid, and she thus frees herself from the complex responsibilities of marriage and child rearing which she finds overwhelming." In partial regression, a person may have some adult thoughts, behaviors, and emotions, but retreats into childlike regression in particular situations.

Joseph Wepman (1962, 1976) suggests that aphasia is a psycholinguistic regression affecting the patient's entire personality (See Chapter 2). For example, the speechlessness of an infant corresponds to global aphasia, semantic aphasia corresponds to the stage of vocabulary learning of a child, syntactic aphasia correlates with the grammatical acquisition stages in children, and so forth. Further, the recovery from aphasia should parallel the stages of language acquisition.

While the "linguistic regression theory" of aphasia has been discounted, some patients with neurogenic communication disorders do regress psychologically. They seek dependent relationships and find comfort in the immature role of a child thus satisfying the need for security. Regression to the immature role of a dependent child may be adaptive and appropriate, particularly during early stages of recovery, especially for severely involved patients. However, because the goal of rehabilitation is to produce an independent and productive individual within the constraints of the neurogenic communication disorder, regression to dependency should be gradually discouraged.

Passive-Aggression

The person engaged in *passive-aggression* appears timid, cautious, and shy, but indirectly expresses his or her anger, hostility, and aggression toward others, particularly authority figures. The passive-aggressive person wants approval and assurance, but as Kolb (1977) observes, timidity masks the underlying hostility. The passive-aggressive person is angry, hostile, and aggressive, but these emotions and behaviors are presented in a passive way.

Patients with neurogenic communication disorders may engage in passive-aggression. For example, a patient with underlying anger, hostility, and aggression may appear to want to fully participate in rehabilitation and agrees to complete therapeutic tasks. However, he or she will not follow through with them. Using the passive-aggressive defense mechanism and coping style, the patient copes with the demands of the neurogenic communication disorder through passive, yet aggressive means. The behavior is seen in dealings with rehabilitation authority figures such as doctors, nurses, and therapists, with whom the patient does not feel comfortable in confronting openly.

Procrastination, lying, making excuses, and complaining are often signs of the passive-aggressive defense mechanism and coping style.

The passive-aggressive defense mechanism and coping style does not require language; it is largely a subconscious process. Thus, language-deprived, global aphasic patients can employ it. Unfortunately, some patients with neurogenic communication disorders, particularly those with frontal lobe syndrome, may be incorrectly deemed passive-aggressive (Tanner and Barnwell, 1994). Lethargy, response-delay, and memory deficits seen in these individuals may resemble passive-aggressive acts.

Reaction Formation

Reaction formation is the substitution of attitudes and behaviors that are diametrically opposed to what the person actually feels and would like to do (Stuart, 2000b). Reaction formation is often seen as excessive behavior, e.g., being too friendly, ordered, cheerful, or generous. "Too much, too often" may signal that a person is engaging in reaction formation in an attempt permanently to relieve anxiety.

Reaction formation may drive a person to be a pornography fighter. The individual may become obsessed with eliminating pornography because it arouses him or her, and anxiety is reduced or eliminated by speaking and writing against it. Although an overused and overgeneralized label, "homophobic' attitudes and behaviors may hide deep-rooted feelings of homosexuality. Freud (1908) considered the trait of cleanliness one manifestation of a reaction formation. In excess, it may be a defense mechanism and coping style against the repressed desire to be messy. Generosity can be a defense against unconscious stinginess, cheerfulness a reaction formation against underlying depression, and engaging in "daredevil" behavior may indicate deep-rooted repressed fears.

All patients with neurogenic communication disorders can use reaction formation including language-deprived persons. For example, a patient who is obsessively orderly may be using reaction formation to deal with deep-seated anxiety associated with the disorganization caused by the disability. Language, which brings order to thought, is lost in global aphasia, and some patients are excessively disturbed by untidy and unkempt hospital rooms and therapy suites. Such behavior can signal attempts by the patient to obtain relief from anxiety associated with environmental disorder. Certainly, not all excessive attitudes and behaviors are reaction formations, but in some patients with neurogenic communication disorders, they can suggest utilization of this defense mechanism and coping style.

Displacement and Projection

Displacement is a subconscious attempt to reduce anxiety by shifting negative emotions from one person or object to another. Usually, the negative emotions are displaced to a neutral or less threatening or dangerous person or object (Stuart, 2001b). Frequently patients and their families direct displacement toward therapists and nurses because doctors are too threatening to confront openly. They may "take out" their anger on the other health care professionals when the source of it is a doctor.

Projection is a subconscious rejection of emotionally unacceptable feelings and thoughts and attributing them to someone else (Stuart, 2001b). In the extreme, delusions and hallucinations are projections of inner turmoil to the outside world. A projecting person subconsciously attributes his or her unacceptable, threatening, and disturbing emotions and thoughts onto someone or something else. Projection reduces anxiety and guilt by blaming others for negative thoughts and emotions.

The patient's family members may sometimes allay anxiety and guilt they may have about their about their inability or unwillingness to care for their loved one by projection. They may project that the members of the rehabilitation team do not provide proper therapies for their loved one, when in reality, the care is appropriate. Statements made by family members, such as "You don't seem to care whether he gets better or not," "You don't spend enough time with my mother," and "You don't put in as much time with my brother as you do with the other patients" may be projections of their own inadequacies. The patient may also indicate that a therapist does not seem motivated to provide quality therapy when, in fact, his or her lack of motivation is being projected to the therapist. Of course, these statements and indications by family members and patients may be accurate appraisals of the situation.

Displacement and projection are capable of being used by language-deprived individuals. Language is not necessary to displace hostility and anger onto a safe person or object. Neither is language necessary to project one's own wishes, motivations, and emotions onto someone else. Both defense mechanisms and coping styles allow the person to avoid awareness of negative thoughts and emotions, and reduce anxiety, by displacing or projecting them.

Altruism, Sublimation, and Substitution

Altruism, sublimation, and *substitution* are categorized together because they involve a person redirecting the negative to personally or socially acceptable thoughts, attitudes, and behaviors. They are similar defense mechanisms and coping styles used to reduce anxiety. Altruism is the attempt to satisfy internal needs by fulfilling the needs of others. Sublimation is the acceptance of a socially approved substitute goal for a drive whose normal mode of expression is blocked (Stuart, 2001b). Substitution is used to reduce anxiety by disguising the motivations for doing something. (Substitution, as used here, does not include the substitution of love objects). When used appropriately, they are mature ways of dealing with negativity and can be used by all patients with neurogenic communication disorders.

An example of altruism is the patient who writes about his or her rehabilitation trials and tribulations. While authors write books for many reasons, books about recovery of illness may be written for altruistic reasons. The patient sublimating aggressive impulses may excel in physical therapy strengthening exercises as a way of venting anger and aggressive impulses. The substituting patient may feel deformed by a stroke or traumatic brain injury, so he or she puts energy into being witty and humorous. The patient who is eager to help others with neurogenic communication disorders may be engaging in an unselfish redirection of negative emotions and drives.

Dissociation

According to Stuart (2001a), *dissociation* is the separation of emotional significance from an idea or situation. It is the detachment of a group of behavioral or mental processes from the rest of the person's consciousness (Stuart, 2001b). Although normal people occasionally dissociate, when done frequently and in excess, it is a radical, desperate attempt to cope with stressors. Dissociation allows the person to remove painful emotions from conscious awareness rather than to feel the pain (Carlat, 1999). There are six types of dissociation: *amnesia, depersonalization, fainting, fugue state, somnambulism,* and *multiple personality.*

As reported previously, organic or psychological factors may cause amnesia. When psychologically based, it is a person's attempt to separate himself or herself from painful information or experience. The selective memory loss relieves anxiety and associated negative emotions associated with the information or experience. Depersonalization can be acute or chronic and, according to Sarason and Sarason (1993), the individual's self-perception changes. It is an altered perception of experience including the sensation that one's identity or some aspect of it is detached from the body. In depersonalization, the person may feel that he or she is an observer looking at the world from above or outside. Fainting is the temporary loss of consciousness and serves as a radical but successful way of dissociating from reality. It is the psychological attempt by the patient to separate himself or herself from the environment. As Eisenson (1984, pp. 187-188) observes, during a catastrophic reaction, a patient may faint: "Vascular changes, irritability, evasiveness, or aggressiveness may precede or accompany the catastrophic reaction. An extreme catastrophic reaction may take the form of loss of consciousness."

> Derealization is sometimes considered a dissociative disorder. It is a person's perception of the world as not being real and that he or she is detached from it.

A fugue state may occur in persons suffering seizures, but when psychologically-based, it is a massive dissociation of personality resulting in the need to seek physical escape. The person in a fugue state may lose identity and become disoriented and confused. Somnambulism is walking while asleep. It is common in children, but in adults, it may be an indication of psychological conflicts. It is associated with dreaming physically active fantasies. Both fugue states and somnambulism require normal physical functions to perform and many patients with neurogenic communication disorders may be unable to engage them. A person with multiple personalities lives two or more lives independently without awareness of the others. Because of the communication barrier in patients with neurogenic communication disorders, discovering whether a person is experiencing multiple personalities is difficult. True multiple personality disorder is rare, and some authorities question whether it exists as a clinical entity.

Defense Mechanisms and Coping Styles Compromised in Aphasia

Because of the loss of language, some defense mechanisms and coping styles are compromised. Global aphasic persons are unable to engage several defense mechanisms and coping styles that require language. *Rationalization and intellectualization, suppression, undoing,* and *humor* are primarily verbal defense mechanisms and coping styles and consequently, more or less, are beyond the capabilities of language-deprived individuals.

Rationalization and Intellectualization

Rationalization and *intellectualization* are often used synonymously as defense mechanisms and coping styles to elevate self-esteem by disguising motivations and masking feelings. However, technically intellectualization is one form of rationalization, excessive reasoning to avoid disturbing emotions (Stuart, 2001a, Stuart, 2001b). It is seeking sanctuary in reason and isolating emotions from an act or behavior.

Rationalization, in the broadest senses, is a conscious attempt by a person to make behaviors and emotions acceptable. It is often considered a face-saving device which relieves guilt and anxiety temporarily. Whether dealing with acts of commission or omission, a person justifies his or her action or inaction by attending to acceptable reasons for them and ignoring or denying unacceptable ones. When rationalization is truthful, and intellectualization based on fact, these attempts by the ego to integrate and accept behaviors and emotions can be mature and adaptive. When used inappropriately, rationalization and intellectualization can restrict functioning and emotional adjustment.

> Rationalization can be both conscious and subconscious processes.

Global aphasic patients, those individuals without language, are impaired or unable to use rationalization and intellectualization. Both defense mechanisms and coping styles are verbal and require language to utilize them. Patients with global aphasia are unable to elevate self-esteem and relieve guilt and anxiety through rationalization and intellectualization.

A patient without language may benefit from *externally imposed rationalization* (Tanner and Barnwell, 1994). During therapy, a clinician can provide rationalization statements in situations where the patient displays anxiety due to poor speech and language performance. Statements made by the clinician such as, "I am sorry, I presented the material too rapidly" and "It is OK, there is too much noise in the room" can help the patient rationalize his or her unsuccessful performance and thus help protect the ego and elevate self-esteem. For externalized rationalizations to be effective, the patient's auditory comprehension must be considered and proper adjustments made to the statements. In addition, externalized rationalizations should be truthful, conducive to ego self-protection, and used sparingly.

Suppression

Suppression, a form of avoidance, is the voluntary exclusion of thoughts from conscious awareness. Negative thoughts, feelings, drives, memories, and ideas are intentionally excluded from the person's consciousness. Patients with neurogenic communication disorders may need to exclude from conscious awareness thoughts, feelings, drives, memories, and ideas related to the verbal impotence they experience because of wordfinding deficits, auditory comprehension impairments, dyslexia, unintelligible speech, and so forth. They may also need to suppress the thoughts associated with loss of the integrity of the self, rejection from others, and the potential of further medical complications and the possibility of death. Unfortunately for global aphasic patients, suppression primarily depends on exercising mental executive control over internal monologues. As a consequence, suppression for language-deprived patients may be ineffective or impossible. In addition, the perseverating patient may find suppression, as an adaptive, mature defense mechanism and coping style, compromised. However, early initiation of treatment may counter the negative effects of perseveration.

Darley (1982, p. 177), in a comprehensive review of the efficacy of aphasia therapy, reports: "Early initiation of treatment results in significantly greater improvement than results when treatment is delayed." While there are many reasons why patients with aphasia benefit more from early rather than delayed treatment, creating a positive mental set early-on may be a major one. Especially in patients with the tendency to perseverate, early initiation of treatment with the support, encouragement, and reinforcements associated with it, may counter the natural tendency to perseverate on the negative.

Undoing

Undoing is an attempt through action or communication to take back an unacceptable behavior or thought. The action or communication is an attempt to partially or completely undo a previous one. Psychologically, the person attempts to deal with emotional conflicts by making amends. It is a subconscious defense mechanism and coping style and a symbolic act (Chisholm, 1993). For example, under stress, a patient may reject a health care professional, engage in profanity, and physically accost him or her. Later, the patient may attempt to undo the previous negative acts by praising the clinician or engaging in more overt attempts to negate the previous actions.

Because undoing is a symbolic act, it is unavailable to global aphasic patients. Global aphasic patients tend to be on a concrete level due to the loss of language (See Chapter 2). Additionally, undoing may be unavailable as a defense mechanism and coping style to language-deprived patients because it requires good communication skills and physical abilities to perform successfully.

Humor

Burgess and Clements (1998) note that with humor, an amusing aspect of a conflict or stressor is emphasized. Prazich (1985, p. 29), a dentist who suffered a cerebral vascular accident with ataxic dysarthria observed: "After a stroke, it is very hard not to be scared and feel sorry for yourself. A very good prescription for both of these feelings is laughter. As a result of losing control of my emotions, I discovered I felt really great inside after a good laugh. I knew this had some actual therapeutic value."

> The appreciation and use of humor as an overt expression of emotions without personal discomfort is a mature psychological defense and coping style (Carlat, 1999).

Most types of humor, with the exception of slapstick and cartoons, require good language skills to appreciate. Many types of humor involve using language in unexpected ways. Consequently, language-deprived patients may be unable to appreciate humor when presented in jokes, monologues, and plays. Humor as a psychological defense and coping style for many global aphasic patients is compromised due to impaired language comprehension and expression. Table 9.2 shows psychological defenses and coping styles and the likelihood of them being compromised in language-deprived patients.

Table 9.2: Psychological Defenses and Coping Styles for Predominantly Internal Threats and Stressors

Psychological Defense and Coping Style	Description	Use by Language-Deprived Patients
Denial	Blocking from conscious awareness of threatening and unpleasant events and situations	Yes
Repression	Excluding from conscious awareness negative thoughts, feelings, drives, memories, and ideas by inhibiting them before or after they reach a conscious level	Yes
Psychological Regression	Retreat to a more secure and comfortable level of adjustment	Yes
Passive-Aggression	Expressing anger, hostility, and aggression toward others in a passive way	Yes

Psychological Defense and Coping Style	Description	Use by Language-Deprived Patients
Reaction Formation	Substitution of attitudes and behaviors that are diametrically opposed to actual ones	Yes
Displacement and Projection	Subconscious attempt to reduce anxiety by shifting negative emotions from one person or object to another or attributing them to someone else	Yes
Altruism, Sublimation, and Substitution	Redirecting the negative to personally or socially acceptable thoughts, attitudes, and behaviors	Yes
Dissociation	Detachment of a group of behavioral or mental processes from the rest of the person's consciousness	Yes, but difficult to determine in some patients with neurogenic communication disorders
Rationalization and Intellectualization	Attempts to elevate self-esteem and avoid disturbing emotions by disguising motivations and masking feelings	Compromised or unavailable
Suppression	Voluntary exclusion of thoughts from conscious awareness	Compromised especially in perseverative patients
Undoing	An attempt through action or communication to take back an unacceptable behavior or thought	Compromised or unavailable
Humor	The appreciation and use of humor as an overt expression of emotions; emphasizing an amusing aspect of a conflict or stressor	Compromised or unavailable

Chapter Summary

Defense mechanisms and coping styles are important in maintaining self-esteem and protection from disturbing emotions, thoughts, and drives. Some are mature and adaptive while others are immature, maladaptive, neurotic, and radical attempts to cope with threats and stressors. Patients use defense mechanisms and coping styles to adjust to the neurogenic communication disorders. Global aphasic patients can use many defense mechanisms and coping styles, but some are compromised or unavailable because they require language. As stressors and threats to self-esteem increase, patients with neurogenic communication disorders may utilize more immature, maladaptive, neurotic, and radical attempts to adjust to them.

Study and Discussion Questions

1. Define and describe defense mechanisms and coping styles.
2. List and discuss the defense mechanisms and coping styles used in threats of a predominantly external nature.
3. Compare and contrast anosognosia and denial.
4. Compare and contrast regression and suppression.
5. What is the "linguistic regression theory" and how does it relate to the defense mechanism and coping style of regression?
6. How might a patient's family project their anxiety and guilt to a health care professional?
7. List and discuss the six types of dissociation.
8. Compare and contrast rationalization and intellectualization.
9. Why does perseveration interfere with suppression?
10. Why are global aphasic patients unable to utilize undoing?
11. Why is language required to engage in humor as a defense mechanism and coping style?
12. List the defense mechanism and coping styles discussed in this chapter in order of their maturity and adaptive value.

References

Boyd, M. (1998). Theoretical basis of psychiatric nursing. In *psychiatric nursing,* M. Boyd and M. Nihart (Eds). Philadelphia: Lippincott.

Burgess, A. and Clements, P. (1998). Stress, coping, and defensive functioning. In *psychiatric nursing,* A. Burgess (Ed). Stamford, CN: Appleton & Lange.

Carlat, D. (1999). *The psychiatric interview.* Philadelphia: Lippincott, Williams & Wilkins.

Carson, R., Butcher, J., and Coleman, J. (1988). *Abnormal psychology and modern life.* Glenview, IL: Foresman and Company.

Chapman, A. (1976). *Textbook of clinical psychiatry,* (2nd ed.). Philadelphia: Lippincott.

Chisholm, M. (1993). Anxiety. In *mental health-psychiatric nursing.* (3rd. ed.). R. Rawlins, S. Williams and C. Beck (Eds). St. Louis: Mosby.

Darley, F.L. (1982). *Aphasia.* Philadelphia: W.B. Saunders.

Eisenson, J. (1984). *Adult aphasia,* (2nd ed.). Englewood Cliffs, NJ: Prentice-Hall.

Freud, S. (1908). *Character and anal erotism.* Standard Edition, Volume 9. London, UK: Hogarth Press.

Kolb, L. (1977). *Modern clinical psychiatry.* Philadelphia: Saunders.

Laraia, M. (1998). Biological context of psychiatric nursing care. In *principles and practice of psychiatric nursing* (6th Ed). G. Stuart and M. Laraia (Eds), St. Louis: Mosby.

Mahl, G. (1971). *Psychological conflict and defense.* New York: Hartcourt Brace Jovanovich.

Millon, T. and Meagher, S. (2004). The millon clinical multiaxial inventory-III (MCMI-III). In *Comprehensive handbook of psychological assessment, Volume 2: Personality assessment.* M. Hilsenroth and D. Segal (Eds). Hoboken, N.J.: John Wiley & Sons.

Porcerelli, J., Thomas, S., Hibbard, S. and Cogan, R. (1998). Defense mechanisms development in children adolescents, and late adolescents. *Journal of Personality Assessment,* 71, 411-420.

Porcerelli, J. and Hibbard, S. (2004). Projective assessment of defense mechanisms. In *Comprehensive handbook of psychological assessment, Volume 2: Personality assessment.* M. Hilsenroth and D. Segal (Eds). Hoboken, N.J.: John Wiley & Sons.

Prazich, M. (1985). *A stroke patient's own story.* Danville, IL: Interstate Printers and Publishers.

Sarason, I. and Sarason, B. (1993). *Abnormal psychology. The problem of maladaptive behavior.* Endglewood Cliffs, NJ: Prentice-Hall.

Stuart, G. (2001a). Self-concept responses and dissociative disorders. In *principles and practice of psychiatric nursing (7ᵗʰ ed.),* G. Stuart and M. Laraia (Eds). St. Louis: Mosby

Stuart, B. (2001b). Anxiety responses and anxiety disorders. In *principles and practice of psychiatric nursing (7ᵗʰ ed.),* G. Stuart and M. Laraia (Eds). St. Louis: Mosby

Tanner, D. and Barnwell, J. (1994). *The psychology of global aphasia. Theoretical and practical issues.* A miniseminar presented to the annual convention of the American Speech-Language-Hearing Association, New Orleans, L.A.

Tanner, D. (2003, Winter). Eclectic perspectives on the psychology of aphasia. *J. Allied Health: 32:256-260.*

Tanner, D. (2009). The psychology of neurogenic communication disorders: A primer for health care professionals. New York: iUniverse.

Wallerstein, R. (1999). *Psychoanalysis: Clinical and theoretical.* Madison, Conn.: International Universities Press.

Wepman, J. (1962). The language disorders. In *Psychological practices with the physically disabled,* J. Garrett and E. Levine (Eds). New York: Columbia University Press.

Wepman, J. (1976). Aphasia: Language without thought or thought without language? *Journal of the American Speech and Hearing Association,* 18: 131-136.

Chapter Ten: The Grief Response

> When you are sorrowful look again
> in your heart, and you shall see that
> in truth you are weeping for that
> which has been your delight.
>
> Kahlil Gibran

Chapter Preview: This chapter examines the grief response in patients with neurogenic communication disorders. Loss of person, self, and object are discussed relative to patients with neurogenic communication disorders. In this chapter, there is a review of the stages many patients with neurogenic communication disorders pass through including a discussion of controversial aspects of the stage model of grief. Grieving denial, response to frustration, grieving depression, and acceptance are reviewed including suggestions to facilitate the patient's resolution of losses.

Neurogenic Communication Disorders and Unwanted Change

On the most basic psychological level, experiencing a neurogenic communication disorder is being subjected to unwanted change. This unwanted change involves loss of valued *persons, aspects of self,* and *valued objects*. Although the patient may not physically lose loved ones because of the neurogenic communication disorder, such as occurs through death, divorce, or separation, impaired or lost speech and language abilities frequently result in social separation from them. Loss of some aspect of self involves the inability or impaired ability to communicate and physical disabilities often co-occurring with neurogenic communication disorders such as walking and swallowing. Because of the communication disorder and physical disabilities, patients can be separated from valued objects such as home, car, pet, garden, library, and other objects with real and symbolic value. Not all neurogenic communication disorders are of the severity to result in significant disabilities for the patient, but many do result in grievous losses and the human reaction to unwanted change - the grief response (Tanner, 2009;Tanner, 2008; Tanner, 2007; Tanner, 2006; Tanner, 2003a; Tanner, 2003b; Tanner and Gerstenberger, 1996; Tanner, 1980). Spillers (2007) and Code, Hemsley, and Herrmann (1999) report the grief model is important to understanding the emotional and psychosocial issues in patients with communication disorders.

Change involving loss occurs throughout a person's life and begins early. The infant loses comfort and security during feedings when he or she is weaned. The birth of another sibling can cause a sense of loss for the only-child. Young adults lose independence and freedom as family and society require more responsibilities. Divorce and separation occur far too often in modern society. People lose valued assets because of untimely investments. Homes and possessions can be lost to fire, theft, and floods. As people age, developmental loss occurs as they lose hearing, sight, attractiveness, physical mobility, and sexual function. And humans are mortal, destined to die, and ultimately lose all worldly connections and life itself. Nevertheless, loss is a natural consequence of living, and so is the grief response. For patients with neurogenic communication disorders, unwanted change is around every corner:

> Loss of self occurs because of loss of the abilities such as walking, talking, dressing, and bowel and bladder control. Loss of person is the psychological separation the patient experiences from family and friends due to the communication disorder, and also because of physical

placement in a nursing home or other type of extended care facility. Loss of object includes the use of a motor home, car, sewing machine, computer, or other valued object or pet due to physical and cognitive limitations and/ or placement in a nursing home" (Tanner, 2007, p. 80).

It is important to emphasize that the sense of loss experienced by patients with neurogenic communication disorders is dependent on their awareness levels. For example, patients with traumatic brain injury or stroke who have reduced or impaired awareness are unlikely to perceive the loss of person, aspect of self, and object to the same extent as someone with intact awareness of his or her situation and predicament. And no one would suggest the grief response occurs in coma or stuporous patients. However, the majority of patients with neurogenic communication disorders are aware of their situation and predicament, suffer significant loss, and can be expected to experience the grief response due to the unwanted changes occurring to them.

> Adjustment to neurogenic communication disorders share similarities with coping with other chronic medical conditions.

Loss of Person

Although the patient does not actually lose his or her loved ones, there can exist a sense of psychological separation due to the neurogenic communication disorder. Grief can result from changes in living arrangements and relationships (Christ, Bonanno, Malkinson, and Rubin, 2003). Because of the communication barriers, the patient may not be able to interact with loved ones as frequently or easily as before. In patients with severe neurogenic communication disorders, especially those with reduced intelligibility and comprehension deficits, the quality of social interaction with significant others can be significantly diminished. Even for patients with mild aphasia, the quality of the relationship with family members may be negatively affected (Parr, 1994). The sense of separation may be increased when patients are confined to long-term medical and rehabilitation facilities.

The real loss of person includes physical separation from loved ones for long periods due to institutionalization and is compounded by the communication barrier. There may also be a symbolic loss. Symbolically, the patient and his or her family may see the neurogenic communication disorder as an insurmountable disability laying waste to what was previously a rich and rewarding relationship. Additionally, in some neurogenic communication disorders, there are sensory deficits which interfere with or prohibit intimate physical contact. In aphasia, the communication disorders crosses all language modalities, more or less, and consequently, also prohibits communication through reading, writing, and complex gestures.

For some patients, the onset of a neurogenic communication disorder may exacerbate preexisting relationship problems. For families having previous relationship problems, the neurogenic communication disorder can perpetuate those troubles and further worsen the relationship. The patient and his or her family may be fixed in the relationship issues with which they were dealing because they can no longer work them out through communication.

> Problems with communication is the number one reason so many marriages fail.

Loss of person as a result of neurogenic communication disorders is both a stressor and barrier to adjusting to the disability. As discussed in Chapter 9, some neurogenic communication disorders are associated with impaired defense mechanisms and coping styles which reduce or eliminate the patient's ability to adjust. Additionally, several psychological reactions and disorders such as emotional lability, catastrophic reactions, perseveration, organic depression-anxiety, anosognosia, homonymous hemianopsia and visual neglect, and euphoria can be precipitated by the brain injury causing the neurogenic communication disorder (See Chapter 8). As a consequence, many patients are subjected to new and unusual stressors, and because of the communicative separation from loved ones, they are deprived of persons with whom they previously would analyze, discuss, and seek counsel about them.

Certainly, not all neurogenic communication disorders are of the severity to result in real and symbolic separation from loved ones. Some neurogenic communication disorders are mild with no appreciable reduction in intelligibility. Others are temporary and patients make complete or near-complete recovery. Never-the-less, many of these neurogenic communication disorders fundamentally disrupt the patient's ability to meaningfully relate to loved ones and impedes relationships with important persons in their lives.

Loss of Some Aspect of Self

Loss of some aspect of self includes unwanted changes in health, body function, sense of worth, self-concept, family role, and perceived attractiveness. It occurs when a person is aware that he or she no longer possesses a previously normal and intact ability or function, and that the loss is irreversible. In patients with neurogenic communication disorders, loss of body function can occur for the ability to communicate, walk, and with several activities of daily living such as dressing, eating, and so forth.

The ability to speak represents potency and patients with severe neurogenic communication disorders can be reduced to near-primitive levels of existence often dramatically affecting their quality-of-life (Tanner, 2003a). Because of the reduced or inability to communicate, many patients' needs, drives, and wishes go unanswered. Expressions of emotions about the patient's predicament can be reduced to nonverbal outbursts often leaving the listener confused about what prompted them.

The loss of language in aphasia can affect the patient's sense of self: "It is possible to experience a sense of being that does not require language. But if a person's knowledge about his/herself is thrown into pure chaos the person may be in need of language to help construe the situation. In some way the aphasic person needs to have a working construct of 'before my illness' versus 'after my illness' and all its implications. Indeed, the grieving process can be viewed as making sense of the construct 'after my illness' and all its implications" (Brumfitt, 1999, p. 352).

The grief response occurs when patients become aware that they are permanently and irreversibly separated from previous valued body functions. The patient recognizes that he or she can no longer function normally. Loss of some aspect of self also includes *developmental loss*, the gradual awareness of unwanted changes due to aging. The onset of a neurogenic communication disorder can bring increased awareness of developmental losses that have occurred for the patient.

Like loss of person, loss of self can have symbolic implications. For example, loss of the ability to walk includes the physical limitations associated with mobility, but also symbolic implications such as lack of freedom and being unable to "stand on one's own two feet." Symbolically, the patient may feel that he or she is relegated to the status of a child because of permanent and irreversible physical losses and is now a dependent ward of his or her family or an institution. Brumfitt (1996) notes that aphasic patients may sense the loss of continuity with the past. They may perceive that independence and mobility are things of days-gone-by. With many patients, there is a *loss of security* and the predictability of usual rewards and punishments. On some level, the patient realizes that life has he or she has known it is unlikely to continue and there is the real threat of another stroke or other devastating medical incident.

Loss of Object

Loss of object includes virtually any external object a person has come to value. The objects people value are highly variable and include home, car, pet, garden, library, computer, recreation vehicle, and so forth. Valued objects are lost to patients with neurogenic communication disorders because of physical and cognitive limitations and disabilities. For example, a patient may lose a recreation vehicle because he or she may be unable to drive or the ability to garden because of confinement to a wheelchair. The motor home may have symbolic value to the person as a representation of the "golden years" of retirement and gardening as a productive use of leisure time. Placement in a long-term medical care facility can cause separation from many valued objects, especially the patient's home and all of the valued object in it. White (2001, p. 309) observes that the significance of the lost object to the individual determines the nature of the grief response: "For instance, an individual who loses a family heirloom in a fire may react not only to the lost financial value of the piece, but also to the lost sense of history and heritage that the piece represented."

> "If you suppress grief too much, it can well redouble." ~Moliere

A patient may lose religious objects when he or she is separated from his or her church. For religious people, being unable to attend church regularly and participate in its rituals can be significant negative consequences of neurological injury. Many religious ceremonies require functional communication abilities, and neurogenic communication disorder can interfere or eliminate a patient's ability to understand and participate in them. There is also the loss of symbols associated with a patient's religion. He or she can be denied the comfort and support they provide.

Accepting Unwanted Change

The grief response is a collection of psychological adjustments a person makes to being permanently separated from something or someone of value. The first and most widely accepted grief model was proposed by Elizabeth Kübler-Ross (1969) in her landmark book, *On Death and Dying*. Kübler-Ross proposed five stages of the grieving process: denial, anger, bargaining, depression, and acceptance. Recently, Kübler-Ross's model has been criticized particularly concerning the order of the stages leading to acceptance. Critics note that not everyone goes through all of the stages and some grieving persons go back and forth between some of them. Actually, Kübler-Ross addressed the order and sequence of the grieving process in her early writings on the subject and noted that the stages and progression are highly variable (Kübler-Ross, 1969). The application of the grief model to the losses experienced by patients with neurogenic communication disorders is also controversial.

Tanner (1980) first proposed the phase model of grief and its application to persons with communication disorders. Tanner and Gerstenberger (1988; 1996) applied the grief model to persons with aphasia. Parr, Byng, Gilpin, and Ireland (1997) examined the grief model concerning aphasic patients using an interview format. They found identifiable stages in aphasic patients but no specific grieving progression through them. According to Lyon and Shadden (2001, p. 302): "Thus, for a majority of Parr et al.'s subjects, there was no evidence of a set coping progression, although anger and denial were typically more prevalent at first, often giving way overtime to some form of internal compromise and/or acceptance. More characteristic, though, was a continuous and overlapping ebb and flow of all of Kübler-Ross's stages, their appearance and reappearance depending on the personal and collective subtleties of those affected."

Although there are several ways of viewing the way patients with neurogenic communication disorders reach acceptance of unwanted changes in their lives, a phase model is useful in describing the grieving process (Boyd, 1998). The phase model is applicable to aware patients with significant and irreversible neurogenic communication disorders with the understanding that not all patients experience all of the stages nor is there always a predictable progression through them. Additionally, in many patients, and their families, friends, and others, there are intermittent bouts of frustration and anger. "For example, one person with aphasia might be 'angry' over the inability to work, 'in denial' about returning to pre-stroke communication levels, and 'accepting' that conversation with family and friends was impractical at the moment" (Lyon and Shadden, 2001, p. 301).

> During grieving, lonely patients may receive attention, support, and contact with others that they would not ordinarily receive. For some patients, these become secondary gains and may cause the patient not to resolve and accept the losses.

Grieving Denial

As noted above, patients with neurogenic communication disorders are likely to experience *denial* when first confronted with irreversible loss of person, some aspect of self, and object. Denial is an early reaction to the loss although the patient may be only partially aware of its irreversibility and permanence. It often occurs initially in the grief response (Parr, Byng, Gilpin, and Ireland, 1997), but can resurface throughout the course of grieving. Some patients may never experience denial and others may chronically engage in it.

Freud (1961) considered denial as a defense mechanism to protect the ego and Kübler-Ross (1969) found it to be an early response to loss. According to Boyd (1998), denial is a stage of shock and disbelief. In denial, the patient may disbelieve what has happened and have an inability to comprehend the implications for his or her life. This defense mechanism and coping style can be characterized by the verbal report, "I do not believe it," made by individuals when initially confronted with the loss of a loved one. Tanner and Gerstenberger (1996) propose four themes of denial in the grief response from a psychiatric perspective: *complete, partial, passive and mystical,* and *existential.* It should be noted that these denial themes may be integral to several other psychological defense mechanisms and coping styles.

In complete denial, the patient believes he or she does not have a disability and often *projects* the communication disorder onto listeners. The patient believes that he or she is talking normally and the communication problems are the result of the listener's inability or unwillingness to understand his or her perfectly normal speech. This type of denial is frequently seen in jargon aphasic patients (Weinstein and Puig-Antich, 1974; Weinstein, Lyerly, Cole, and Ozer, 1966). As discussed in Chapters 3 and 9, denial is associated with specific brain lesions, but it is also at least partially related to the patients need to protect his or her ego from anxiety and awareness of grievous losses. This statement summarizes complete denial and projection from the perspective of the patient: "I do not have a speech-language disorder and the communication problem is the result of the listener's inability or unwillingness to understand my perfectly normal speech."

Patients in partial denial may have awareness of some aspect of loss but deny others. For example, a patient may be aware of loss of self concerning the ability to speak, but denies the implications of impaired communication on his or her relationships. Patients may also minimize the losses, believe they are temporary, or otherwise deny the totality of what has happened to them. Partial denial from the perspective of the patient can be summarized by this statement: "I have a communication disorder but it is minor, temporary, and/or insignificant."

Patients with an external frame of reference may present with denial having a passive and mystical theme. The patient is at least partially aware that he or she has a communication disorder, but is certain that external forces will accomplish complete recovery. The patient denies the reality of the communication disorder and is usually passive about rehabilitation. He or she may direct his or her energies to prayer and faith healing rituals. "I have a significant neurogenic communication disorder, but it is temporary and God will make me whole again" summarizes the patient with a passive and mystical denial theme.

In contrast to patients with an external frame of reference, denial with an existential theme involves a person's belief in the ability to overcome completely a neurogenic communication disorder through will and determination. These patients have an internal frame of reference. LaPointe (1997) found that patients who have an internal locus of control do better with adjustment to aphasia. Denial with an existential theme is only partial because the patient acknowledges the neurogenic communication disorder, but is unrealistic about his or her ability to overcome it. This statement summarizes denial with an existential theme: "I have a neurogenic communication disorder but through my will and determination, I will overcome it and return to complete normalcy."

> Arthur Kopit wrote the Broadway Play, *Wings*, about a person with aphasia. The play captures the isolation and desolation of aphasia. It was commissioned by National Public Radio and released in 1978.

Denial is a lower order defense mechanism and coping style not requiring language and is readily available to patients deprived of language. Denial should be distinguished from misinformation. A patient in denial has been provided with accurate and complete information about the neurogenic communication disorder, yet denies all or part of it. The misinformed patient has not been accurately and completely apprised of his or her predicament. No matter the theme of the denial, it serves to prevent anxiety and buffer psychological pain. Denial permits the patient to avoid confrontation with the losses associated with the neurogenic communication disorder. Denial as an unrealistic positive view about disabilities can, in many instances, be congruent with mental health (Telford, Kralik, and Koch, 2005). At the very least, it allows the patient the time and opportunity to mobilize less radical defenses.

Encouraging and rewarding denial in the grieving patient should be avoided. As reported above, denial is an extreme defense mechanism and coping style requiring a great deal of psychological energy. A less radical buffer to psychological pain should replace it as soon as possible. Of course, brutal confrontation of denial should also be avoided because it can push the patient, and his or her family and friends, deeper into it. Counselors working with terminally ill patients know that most patients move from denial into more productive stages when their needs dictate it. Clinicians working with denying patients should provide a degree of hope when giving prognoses for recovery from neurogenic communication disorders. However, if the patient persists in denial, referral to a psychiatrist, psychologist, or counselor is indicated.

Response to Frustration

Many patients with neurogenic communication disorders are frustrated by their attempts to overcome losses and *anger* and *bargaining* are natural, normal reactions to that frustration. Anger and bargaining are expected reactions on the part of the patient to the loss of control that arises from two sources. First, the patient is generally frustrated by the inability to alter the course of events leading to the losses and the unwanted changes in his or her life. There are many unalterable realities surrounding the brain and nervous system damage, and the patient is frustrated in his or her ability to change or eliminate them. Second, the patient may be frustrated by the inability to communicate with others normally. Although some neurogenic communication disorders are not frustrating, many are. There can be frustration associated with auditory comprehension, word finding, speech programming, and attempts to produce intelligible speech. Reading, writing, and simple arithmetic may also be significantly impaired rendering the patient frustratingly unable to perform them as he or she once did easily. The chronic inability to consummate the communication act can be extremely frustrating and anger-provoking for some patients.

The anger felt by many patients with neurogenic communication disorders can take several forms. Some patients are passive in their anger and express it by missing appointments, isolating themselves from others, refusing treatment, and so forth. Other patients express anger by striking out at health care professionals, family, and friends. Angry patients with functional speech may use profanity and denigrate others.

Nonverbal patients may inwardly direct anger and feel guilt for their predicament. Some authorities believe this inward direction of anger causes depression. According to Carlat (1999), anger may be related to irritability associated with depression, and Chisholm (1993) observes that frustration may lead to depression. Frustration leads to anger, and the inner direction of anger can bring on depression in some patients with neurogenic communication disorders.

Anger is a natural and normal reaction to the frustration associated with grievous losses. Consequently, in most situations, it should neither be punished nor discouraged. However, if the anger displayed by the patient is destructive to himself or herself, or to others, then intervention is necessary. It is important that the patient understand that it is not the expression of anger that is being discouraged, only the inappropriate manner in which negative emotions are being ventilated. Exercise and other strenuous activities are constructive methods of dealing with anger. The patient can also be provided with a harmless object that can be used for symbolic ventilation of emotions. Of course, with patients who are chronically angry, a psychiatric referral may be necessary.

> According to LaPointe (1997), favorable pre-injury personality tendencies having a positive influence on coping with neurogenic communication disorders include adaptability, persistence, attentiveness, and pleasant and stable moods.

Bargaining, another reaction to frustration, is the attempt by the patient to reduce or delay the losses. The patient offers some good behavior, or seeks help from a higher authority, to reduce, postpone, or eliminate the unwanted changes in his or her life. Bargaining patients may do so with themselves, family members, and God. Bargaining may also occur with health care professionals. In the bargain, the patient turns over the disorder to higher authorities. Similar to denial, bargaining allows the patient to postpone becoming completely aware of what has been taken from him or her.

While bargaining with health care professionals may be nonverbal, it can be summarized in this statement: "If I enthusiastically participate in rehabilitation, and do everything required of me, I will get complete return of my abilities." The patient focuses on complete recovery of lost abilities and his or her frustration is reduced because he or she believes the bargain. A positive aspect of bargaining is that the patient may be highly motivated and responsive to rehabilitation. Of course, health care professionals should avoid being unrealistic with patients about the value and outcomes of therapeutic services. Providing false hope during the bargaining stage may perpetuate bargaining, and although the patient may be highly motivated, it is based on an unrealistic assessment that he or she will make complete recovery. The patient may require more of himself or herself than is desirable and practical, and will ultimately be disappointed. In some instances, the patient may be fixated in bargaining and never reach acceptance of his or her losses.

Health care professionals can reduce the frustration patients experience about the unwanted changes occurring in their lives by providing them with as much control as possible. Many decisions made in rehabilitation *for* the patient can be made *by* them. For example, many patients can and should be active participants in setting treatment goals and the procedures used to obtain them. Most importantly to reducing frustration during therapies, patients should succeed more than they fail. Clinicians should carefully design treatments to ensure that unobtainable goals do not unnecessarily frustrate patients. Carefully redefining the steps necessary to achieve an objective can accomplish this. Additionally, each session should begin and end with successful performance by the patient.

For grieving patients who are frustrated by their neurogenic communication disorders, special efforts should be taken to reduce the inherent frustration associated with speech production. By word or deed, clinicians should communicate to these patients that they cannot "force" speech to be produced correctly. Trial and error strategies are the best methods for word finding and speech programming and execution. Particularly with apraxia of speech, forcing speech increases propositionality which decreases the accuracy of motor speech programming (See Chapter 5). In addition, with most patients, speech "perfection" is an unnecessary and unobtainable goal. The inherent frustration in neurogenic communication disorders can be reduced by recognizing that speech production need not be perfect to consummate communication.

Sometimes patients with neurogenic communication disorders will attempt to communicate something apparently important to their family, friends, and health care professionals, but are impotent in doing so. These often become frustrating "games of Charades." In those incidences where it is clear that the patient's thoughts will not be forthcoming, listeners should minimize the frustration associated with the verbal impotence. This can be done by communicating to the patient that the listener considers the information important, but because of the frustrating impediment, it will be returned to at a later date. This strategy does not negate the importance of what the patient intends to say; it does however, bring an end the frustrating attempt to communicate it, at least temporarily.

Grieving Depression

Grieving depression occurs in patients with neurogenic communication disorders who are aware they have suffered significant losses. It is a natural, predictable result of permanent separation from valued persons, aspects of self, and valued objects. Patients with neurogenic communication disorders may become depressed when they no longer deny the losses, feel anger about them, and realize bargaining will no longer prevent them. During grieving depression, the patient appreciates the full value of what has been lost. Losses that are less significant to the patient will produce less depression than those losses that are of greater value.

Although depression can occur at any stage in the grieving process and reappear throughout it, patients become depressed when all other attempts to overcome the losses have failed. The duration of normal grieving depression may range from only a few days to several months, and some patients may become chronically depressed. Bouts of grieving depression may be triggered by stimuli for months and even years after the losses.

Normal grieving depression is also associated with chemical changes occurring in the brain described in Chapter 8, but it is reactive and proportional to the losses experienced by the patient. This type of depression is also independent of the hemisphere, site, and size of the brain lesion. Grieving depression is not simply a biochemical deficiency induced prolonged feeling of sadness, hopelessness, anxiety, and helplessness. Of course, both organic and reactive depression may occur in some patients. "Early on, for example, structural neurobiochemical changes within the brain, depending on the size and location of lesion, may dominate emotional stability. Later on, when the biochemistry of the brain has either stabilized or been augmented through antidepressant medications, reactive 'blues' in response to lasting functional losses may emerge as more influential" (Lyon and Shadden, 2001, p. 302). If the depression follows a period of bargaining and high levels of cooperation in rehabilitation, during depression, there may be a dramatic drop in the patient's motivation levels.

> Studies show that family members report more negative emotions in stroke patients than self-reported by the patients and aphasic patients tend to show little concern about or awareness of caregiver depression (Lyon and Shadden, 2001).

Grieving depression may also be psychotic and accompanied by mania and agitation (Tanner and Gerstenberger, 1996). These psychotic episodes may be the result of the patient returning to denial. "Persistent euphoria and mania, however, signal regression to radical defences and/or psycho-organic deficits symptomatic of psychotic depression" (Tanner and Gerstenberger, 1996, p. 317). Grieving depression should not be considered abnormal when it is appropriate to the losses experienced by the patient. Patients should be provided opportunities to grieve privately and time set aside for that purpose. Toward the later stages of the grief response, being immersed in rehabilitation, work, or a hobby may be beneficial. However, overindulgence in activities and too early distractions may cause depression to deepen. Patients need to be able to be fully aware of the losses they have experienced.

The overall suicide rate is 10.9 deaths per 100,000 people (National Institute of Mental Health, 2007). However, some authorities believe this is a low estimate due to under-reporting, and many more depressed persons attempt suicide. In grieving depression, suicide is the result of the patient wanting to avoid and escape the realities of the losses and the depression. According to the National Institute of Mental Health (2007), the suicide rate is also higher in the elderly. Because of the higher risk of suicide, clinicians should be alert to signs of it including a family history of suicide, reports, and previous attempts.

Resolution and Acceptance

The goal of the grief response is *resolution* and *acceptance* of the losses. Usually acceptance is the final stage of the grieving process, but it may be partial or complete. A patient may be accepting about one aspect of the losses he or she has suffered, but not accepting of another (Lyon and Shadden, 2001). Additionally, some accepting patients may return to previous aspects of the grief response when triggered by stimuli or general stress.

Resolution and acceptance are not the same as *resignation* to the losses suffered by the patient with a neurogenic communication disorder. Resignation implies that the patient tolerates the losses and the despair associated with them. In resignation, the patients psychologically surrenders to the unwanted changes in his or her life. Resignation to the losses is reflected in this statement: "I have suffered terrible losses, but there is nothing I can do about the situation, so I will tolerate them." Resolution and acceptance, on the other hand, means the patient feels neither good nor bad about what has been lost and he or she is often void of emotions about them. In resolution and acceptance, the patient has assimilated the losses into a larger psychological framework.

Patients with neurogenic communication disorders who have resolved and accepted their losses remain good rehabilitation candidates. In fact, many patients are more realistically motivated to improve their communication abilities and have more energy to do so. They can redirect their energies to rehabilitation because they are no longer attempting to psychologically prevent their losses and are no longer depressed. They continue to strive for improvement.

> "Treatments for the consequences of aphasia's chronicity are only in their infancy, and are diverse in their form, purpose, setting, and type of participation. It seems likely that we will find that no single means of management, (group, dyadic, or individual) or single participant (person with aphasia, significant other, family, friend, employer, or stranger) is sufficient to return disrupted life systems to preferred or optimal states of wellness" (Lyon and Shadden, 2001 p. 304).

Health Care Professionals and the Grieving Patient

Understanding the process of grieving is beneficial to health care professionals when dealing with patients with neurogenic communication disorders (Keller, Tanner, Urbina, and Gerstenberger, 1989). Whether the health care professional believes that grieving is a series of phases a patient passes through, or that grief is a collection of relatively independent psychological reaction, he or she can do and say things that facilitate or interrupt the patient's eventual resolution and acceptance of losses.

One of the most important things a health care professional can do to facilitate the patient's resolution and acceptance of his or her losses is to provide him or her with perspective about the grief response. Many patients in the acute stages of grieving may believe there will never be an end to the cycle of loss and psychological pain and sorrow he or she is experiencing. Perspective can be given to grieving patients by explaining that what he or she is going through is finite and there will be an end to it. Patients should be made aware that there is "light at the end of the tunnel" in the form of resolution and acceptance. Of course, communicating this to patients with severely impaired speech and language abilities is challenging. One way of giving patients a positive perspective is to have a well-adjusted past patient meet with the griever. By seeing someone who has successfully resolved and accepted his or her losses, the patient will gain a positive perspective.

Support groups also can be valuable in giving grieving patients a positive perspective.

For many grieving patients, health care professionals may be considered "detached observers" and they may open-up more readily to them than with family and friends. They may talk more freely and discuss sensitive loss issues with clinicians than with persons with whom they have established relationships. Grieving patients may not want to discuss their fears and anxieties with children and spouses so as to maintain previous roles. Health care professionals can provide valuable support during grieving by simply being sympathetic listeners. However, Telford, Kralik, and Koch (2005) note that health care professionals who adopt the stage theory of grieving may not attentively listen when patients with chronic illnesses relate their unique stories about coping with their illnesses.

When interacting with the grieving patient, clinicians should avoid trying to "make it all right" by uttering a statement. No matter how well-intentioned, these statements can be perceived as being flippant. There is simply no statement that can be made to do away with the psychological pain and sorrow for the bereaved patient. Similarly, providing a religious philosophy may be well-intentioned and helpful if the patient shares the same religious philosophy. However, even in these situations, it is better to leave religious discussions to the patient's family, friends, and religious leaders. Table 10.1 shows the dimensions of loss, stages of resolution and acceptance, and suggestions to health care professionals in facilitating the grieving process.

Table 10.1: Dimensions of Loss, Psychological Reactions, and Factors Facilitating and Interrupting the Grieve Response

Dimension of Loss	Reaction to Unwanted Changes	Factors Facilitating the Grief Response	Factors Interrupting the Grief Response
Person	Grieving denial	Permit the patient control	Rewarding and encouraging denial
Some aspect of self	Response to frustration: Anger Bargaining	Provide a realistic perspective	Contributing to frustration
Object	Grieving depression	Acknowledge the reality of the losses	Bargaining with the patient
Developmental loss Loss of security	Resolution and acceptance	Sympathetic listening	Providing too early distractions and interrupting private grief

Chapter Summary

There comes a time when patients must cease attempting to overcome neurogenic communication disorders and focus attention to resolving and accepting the permanent unwanted changes in their lives. Neurogenic communication disorders are associated with real and symbolic losses of persons, aspects of self, and valued objects. Many patients experience grieving denial, frustration, grieving depression, and eventual resolution and acceptance of the losses they have experienced. While many patients pass through predictable stages leading to resolution and acceptance of the losses associated with neurogenic communication disorders, others have similar but relatively independent psychological reactions. Health care professionals can be important in facilitating the grieving process to help patients eventually resolve and accept their losses.

Study and Discussion Questions

1. Describe how neurogenic communication disorder may cause real and symbolic separation from valued persons.

2. What are the aspects of self that can be lost to patients with neurogenic communication disorders?

3. Describe developmental loss and loss of security as they pertain to neurogenic communication disorders.

4. List and discuss the objects of value in your life and how neurogenic communication disorders might result in their loss.

5. Describe and criticize the phase model of the grief response.

6. Describe the themes of grieving denial described by Tanner and Gerstenberger (1996).

7. What are the typical responses to frustration experienced by patients with neurogenic communication disorders? Describe them.

8. When should anger be discouraged or punished in a grieving patient?

9. Compare and contrast grieving and psycho-organic depression.

10. Describe resolution and acceptance of neurogenic communication disorders.

11. What can health care professionals do to facilitate the patient's reaching of resolution and acceptance of his or her losses?

12. How can health care professionals avoid interrupting the patient's resolution and acceptance of his or her losses?

References

Boyd, M. (1998). Biopsychosocial aspects of stress and crisis. In *Psychiatric nursing,* M. Boyd and M. Nihart (Eds). Philadelphia: Lippincott.

Brumfitt, S. (1996). Losing your sense of self: What aphasia can do. In *Forums in clinical aphasiology,* C. Code (Ed). London: Whurr Publishers.

Carlat, D. (1999). *The psychiatric interview.* Philadelphia: Lippincott, Williams & Wilkins.

Chisholm, M. (1993). Anxiety. In *mental health-psychiatric nursing.* (3rd. ed.). R. Rawlins, S. Williams, and C. Beck (Eds). St. Louis: Mosby.

Christ, G., Bonanno, G., Malkinson, R., and Rubin, S. (2003). Bereavement experiences after the death of a child. When children die: Improving palliative and end-of-life care for children and their families. Washington, DC: *National Academy Press*; pp. 553-579.

Code, C., Hemsley, G., and Herrmann, M. (1999). The emotional impact of aphasia. *Seminars in speech and language,* Volume 20, Number 1, pp. 19-31.

Freud, S. (1961). *The ego and the id: Standard edition of the complete psychological works of Freud,* Vol XIX. London: Hogarth Press.

Keller, C., Tanner, D., Urbina, C., and Gerstenberger, D. (1989). Psychological responses in aphasia: Theoretical considerations and nursing implications. *Journal of Neuroscience Nursing.* October, Vol. 21, No. 5: 290-294.

Kübler-Ross, E. (1969). *On death and dying.* New York: Macmillan.

LaPointe, L.L. (1997). Adaptation, accommodation, aristos. In L. L. LaPointe, *Aphasia and related neurogenic language disorders* (2nd ed.). New York: Thieme.

Lyon, J. and Shadden, B. (2001). Treating life consequences of aphasia's chronicity. In *Language intervention in aphasia and related neurogenic communication disorders* (4th ed.). R. Chapey (Ed). Philadelphia: Lippincott Williams and Wilkins.

National Institute of Mental Health (2007). Suicide in the U.S.: statistics and prevention. Retrieved from the World Wide Web October 14, 2007: http://www.nimh.nih.gov/health/publications/ suicide-in-the-us-statistics-and-prevention.shtml

Parr, S, Byng, S., Gilpin, S. and Ireland, C. (1997). *Talking about aphasia*. Philadelphia: Open University Press.

Parr, S. (1994). Coping with aphasia. Conversations with 20 aphasic people. *Aphasiology*, 8(5): 457-466.

Spillers, C. (2007, August). An existential framework for understanding the counseling needs of clients. *American Journal of Speech-Language Pathology*, Vol.16: 191-197.

Tanner, D. (1980). Loss and grief: Implications for the speech-language pathologist and audiologist. *Journal of the American Speech and Hearing Association*, 22:916-928.

Tanner, D. (2003, Winter). Eclectic perspectives on the psychology of aphasia. *J. Allied Health: 32:256-260.*

Tanner, D. (2006). *Case studies in communication sciences and disorders.* Upper Saddle River, N.J.: Pearson Merrill Prentice Hall.

Tanner, D. (2007). *Medical-legal and forensic aspects of communication disorders, voice prints, and speaker profiling.* Tucson: Lawyers and Judges Publishing.

Tanner, D. (2008). *The family guide to surviving stroke and communication disorders* (2nd ed.). Sudbury, M.A.: Jones and Bartlett.

Tanner, D. (2009). *The psychology of neurogenic communication disorders: A primer for health care professionals.* New York: iUniverse.

Tanner, D. and Gerstenberger, D. (1988). The grief response in neuropathologies of speech and language. *Aphasiology*, 1 (6):79-84.

Tanner, D. and Gerstenberger, D. (1996). Clinical Forum 9: The grief model in aphasia. In *Forums in clinical aphasiology*, C. Code (Ed). London: Whurr Publishers

Telford, K., Kralik, D. and Koch, T. (2005). Acceptance and denial: Implications for people adapting to chronic illness: Literature review. *Journal of Advanced Nursing* 55 (4), 457–464.

Weinstein, E., Lyerly, O., Cole, M., and Ozer, M. (1966). Meaning in Jargon aphasia. *Cortex*, 2: 165-187.

Weinstein, E. and Puig-Antich, J. (1974). Jargon and its analogues. *Cortex*, 10:75-83.

White, L. (2001). *Foundations of nursing: Caring for the whole person.* Albany, N.Y.: Delmar Thompson Learning.

www.ingramcontent.com/pod-product-compliance
Lightning Source LLC
Chambersburg PA
CBHW031819170526
45157CB00001B/111